GETTING THE BEST FOR YOUR BAD BACK

ANTHONY CAMPBELL MRCP is an NHS Consultant Physician at the Royal London Homoeopathic Hospital, fellow of the Faculty of Homoeopathy and member of the British Medical Acupuncture Society. He has taught acupuncture to doctors for many years. Much of his work involves the treatment of back problems. He is the author of books on alternative medicine and Indian philosophy.

GW00597222

Overcoming Common Problems Series

For a full list of titles please contact
Sheldon Press, Marylebone Road, London NW1 4DU

Beating Job Burnout
DR DONALD SCOTT

Beating the Blues
SUSAN TANNER AND JILLIAN BALL

Being the Boss
STEPHEN FITZSIMON

Birth Over Thirty
SHEILA KITZINGER

Body Language
How to read others' thoughts by their gestures
ALLAN PEASE

Bodypower
DR VERNON COLEMAN

Bodysense
DR VERNON COLEMAN

Calm Down
How to cope with frustration and anger
DR PAUL HAUCK

Changing Course
How to take charge of your career
SUE DYSON AND STEPHEN HOARE

Comfort for Depression
JANET HORWOOD

Complete Public Speaker
GYLES BRANDRETH

Coping Successfully with Your Child's Asthma
DR PAUL CARSON

Coping Successfully with Your Hyperactive Child
DR PAUL CARSON

Coping Successfully with Your Irritable Bowel
ROSEMARY NICOL

Coping with Anxiety and Depression
SHIRLEY TRICKETT

Coping with Blushing
DR ROBERT EDELMANN

Coping with Cot Death
SARAH MURPHY

Coping with Depression and Elation
DR PATRICK McKEON

Coping with Stress
DR GEORGIA WITKIN-LANOIL

Coping with Suicide
DR DONALD SCOTT

Coping with Thrush
CAROLINE CLAYTON

Curing Arthritis – The Drug-Free Way
MARGARET HILLS

Curing Arthritis Diet Book
MARGARET HILLS

Curing Coughs, Colds and Flu – The Drug-Free Way
MARGARET HILLS

Curing Illness – The Drug-Free Way
MARGARET HILLS

Depression
DR PAUL HAUCK

Divorce and Separation
ANGELA WILLANS

Don't Blame Me!
How to stop blaming yourself and other people
TONY GOUGH

The Epilepsy Handbook
SHELAGH McGOVERN

Everything You Need to Know about Adoption
MAGGIE JONES

Everything You Need to Know about Contact Lenses
DR ROBERT YOUNGSON

Everything You Need to Know about Osteoporosis
ROSEMARY NICOL

Overcoming Common Problems Series

Everything You Need to Know about Shingles
DR ROBERT YOUNGSON

Everything You Need to Know about Your Eyes
DR ROBERT YOUNGSON

Family First Aid and Emergency Handbook
DR ANDREW STANWAY

Feverfew
A traditional herbal remedy for migraine and arthritis
DR STEWART JOHNSON

Fight Your Phobia and Win
DAVID LEWIS

Getting Along with People
DIANNE DOUBTFIRE

Getting Married
JOANNA MOORHEAD

Goodbye Backache
DR DAVID IMRIE WITH COLLEEN DIMSON

Heart Attacks – Prevent and Survive
DR TOM SMITH

Helping Children Cope with Divorce
ROSEMARY WELLS

Helping Children Cope with Grief
ROSEMARY WELLS

Helping Children Cope with Stress
URSULA MARKHAM

Hold Your Head Up High
DR PAUL HAUCK

How to be a Successful Secretary
SUE DYSON AND STEPHEN HOARE

How to Be Your Own Best Friend
DR PAUL HAUCK

How to Control your Drinking
DRS W. MILLER AND R. MUNOZ

How to Cope with Stress
DR PETER TYRER

How to Cope with Tinnitus and Hearing Loss
DR ROBERT YOUNGSON

How to Cope with Your Child's Allergies
DR PAUL CARSON

How to Cure Your Ulcer
ANNE CHARLISH AND DR BRIAN GAZZARD

How to Do What You Want to Do
DR PAUL HAUCK

How to Get Things Done
ALISON HARDINGHAM

How to Improve Your Confidence
DR KENNETH HAMBLY

How to Interview and Be Interviewed
MICHELE BROWN AND GYLES BRANDRETH

How to Love a Difficult Man
NANCY GOOD

How to Love and be Loved
DR PAUL HAUCK

How to Make Successful Decisions
ALISON HARDINGHAM

How to Move House Successfully
ANNE CHARLISH

How to Pass Your Driving Test
DONALD RIDLAND

How to Say No to Alcohol
KEITH McNEILL

How to Spot Your Child's Potential
CECILE DROUIN AND ALAIN DUBOS

How to Stand up for Yourself
DR PAUL HAUCK

How to Start a Conversation and Make Friends
DON GABOR

How to Stop Smoking
GEORGE TARGET

How to Stop Taking Tranquillisers
DR PETER TYRER

How to Stop Worrying
DR FRANK TALLIS

How to Study Successfully
MICHELE BROWN

Overcoming Common Problems Series

Overcoming Common Problems

GETTING THE BEST FOR YOUR BAD BACK

Dr Anthony Campbell

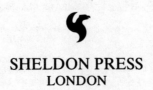

SHELDON PRESS
LONDON

First published in Great Britain 1992
Sheldon Press, SPCK, Marylebone Road, London NW1 4DU

Illustrations by Alasdair Smith

British Library Cataloguing-in-Publication Data
A catalogue record for this book is available from the British Library

ISBN 0–85969–651–0

Photoset by Deltatype Ltd, Ellesmere Port, Cheshire
Printed in Great Britain by Biddles Ltd, Guildford and King's Lynn

Contents

Introduction

Disorders of the back are among the commonest ills that afflict human beings. No fewer than 80 per cent of us can expect to suffer at least one episode of back pain during our active lives, and back disorders are among the commonest causes of absence from work.

Back pain can take many forms. A young person may suffer a 'stiff neck' on waking one morning: it comes on suddenly, for no apparent reason, and disappears as mysteriously after a few days; a middle-aged man digs his garden one Sunday in spring, and wakes up next morning to find his lower back stiff and painful, recognizing what has happened because he has suffered from 'lumbago' before; a woman loads shopping into her car, twisting her back awkwardly as she does so, and that evening experiences a dull ache in the lower part of her back, which persists all the following day. On the second morning she wakes to find that her back is so stiff that she cannot put on her shoes and she is in constant severe pain. Later the pain eases somewhat in her back but instead she begins to experience severe pain in her leg – sciatica; a fit young man of thirty bends forwards to pick up something from the ground and suddenly his back 'locks', so that he cannot move or straighten himself.

These are just some of the ways that back pain may occur. But in spite of the importance of the problem, it is surprisingly difficult to get firm answers to the question of why it occurs. We are sometimes told that the ultimate cause is our 'unnatural' upright stance; if we walked on all fours, the argument runs, we would not suffer from back problems. But this isn't very plausible.

For one thing, quadrupeds do in fact suffer from back disorders: dogs and race horses, for example, certainly do; nor is it only modern domesticated animals that are affected: changes typical of spinal degeneration have been found in fossils of dinosaurs. For another, our species and its immediate ancestors have walked upright for at least 2 million years, probably longer, so it is unlikely that our skeletal system has not adapted to the posture by now.

It is claimed, too, that the incidence of back pain is increasing, but this argument, also, is hard to sustain. We cannot know for certain how frequent the complaint was in former times, but skeletons from Egyptian tombs and Saxon burials, for instance, show changes that indicate the existence of disease of the spine. Probably things are much the same today as they were in the past.

Although we still know very little about the mechanisms of pain in many cases of back pain, this ignorance should not be overstated; some things at least have become clear. Until quite recently (within the last fifty years), for example, doctors didn't realize that the pain of sciatica was, in many cases, caused by an intervertebral disc compressing a nerve root. New methods of investigating the living spine, such as computerized (axial) tomographic (CT or CAT) and magnetic resonance imaging (MRI) (see p. 53) scanning, are providing much more information about what goes wrong with the back mechanically. At the same time, however, a great deal of treatment is still 'empirical'; that is, it seems to work but no one is quite sure why.

To the average backache sufferer it may seem that an answer to the question 'Why have I got this pain?' should be reasonably easy to obtain. Having examined the patient, and perhaps taken an X-ray, the doctor ought to be able to say what is wrong – a 'slipped disc', perhaps or a 'trapped nerve' – without too much trouble, surely. After all, the back is a physical structure – more complex than a car engine, no doubt, but in principle still capable of being understood in the same mechanical terms, so why are satisfactory explanations for back pain not always forthcoming?

There are several reasons. First, there is the plain fact that there are still many things we don't know about the structure and function of the back. (The same is of course true of every other part of the body.) Second, there is the sheer complexity of the back as a structure: it forms the core of the body, supporting the head and trunk. Because of its central position, almost anything that affects any other part of the body may have a secondary, indirect effect on the back as well. Sorting out all these influences is often difficult or even impossible. Moreover, the back is a mechanical system, certainly, but one that contains a huge number of components – muscles, bones, ligaments, nerves – whose structure and function, to say nothing of their interactions, are only partially understood. It is hardly ever justifiable to isolate one component and then say that it is the sole cause of a patient's symptoms. An X-ray, for example, may show that a pair of adjacent vertebrae in someone complaining of back pain have ceased to move normally on each other because of disease. But this may not be what is causing the pain; the source of discomfort may be the vertebral joints further up which are moving excessively in order to compensate for the fixity below.

It is not just a matter of the mechanical complexity of the spine that makes simplistic explanations inadequate. We also have to consider the issue of *how* pain is felt and perceived and this, too, is a more complicated subject than is sometimes realized.

For all these reasons, self-diagnosis of back pain, especially when it is a first attack, is not advisable. The best person to see in the first instance is nearly always your family doctor. So far as specialist advice is concerned, you might need the help of a neurologist, an orthopaedic surgeon, a gynaecologist, a general physician, a physiotherapist, or even a psychiatrist, to say nothing of the numerous practitioners of complementary medicine such as acupuncture and osteopathy. Your family doctor is the best person to help you orientate yourself in this therapeutic maze and to point you in the right direction if he or she is not able to help you enough.

No one practitioner can be familiar in practice with every kind of treatment that may be used for back pain; the range of possible approaches is too wide for this. My own background is that of an orthodoxly trained doctor with a special interest in two forms of complementary treatment, acupuncture and homoeopathy. As a consultant physician at The Royal London Homoeopathic Hospital I see many patients with back pain, and the hospital provides a number of different treatments for this complaint. These include not only acupuncture and homoeopathy but also, if appropriate, manipulation, relaxation, and autogenic training (a more elaborate form of relaxation); conventional medicine is also used if necessary, and patients may be referred to other hospitals for possible surgery if that seems most likely to help.

In practice, acupuncture is usually our first treatment choice for back pain, and it provides at least a fair measure of relief for about 70 per cent of the patients we see. However, each patient is assessed individually, and the decision about which form of treatment to try is based not only on the objective findings but also in part on the patient's preference.

1

Structure and Function

This chapter describes the anatomy of the back and may seem somewhat dry. If you find it so, you may prefer to go straight on to Chapter 2, coming back to this one from time to time as necessary to clarify your understanding of particular topics. The Glossary (see p. 105) also provides brief explanations of anatomical and other terms and is useful for quick reference.

The back is a complex structure made up of a number of components. At its core, so to speak, there are the bones and joints, which are held together by ligaments (bands of fibre-rich tissue). Together, these components constitute the spine proper. Surrounding the bones and joints and ligaments are the muscles, which serve both to move the back and also to support it and maintain its structural integrity. Other important components include blood vessels and nerves.

The spine consists of 26 bones: 24 vertebrae (sing. vertebra), the sacrum, and the tiny vestigial tail, the 'coccyx', which is made up of four small vertebrae fused together. On top of the spine sits the skull. It exerts considerable leverage on the whole structure because it is heavy. (See Figure 1.)

There are five main zones of the spine, each with its own characteristics. The neck (cervical) region, with 7 vertebrae, is the most mobile. The chest (thoracic) region has 12 vertebrae and provides attachment for the ribs and the upper limbs. The back (lumbar) region has 5 vertebrae and is thick and strong, and relatively immobile because it has to carry all the weight of the upper half of the body. The sacrum – a wedge-shaped bone at the base of the lumbar region and composed of 5 vertebrae fused together – plus the coccyx, form the back of the pelvis, to which the lower limbs are attached. The pelvis needs to be particularly strong and rigid in a species like ours which walks on its hind limbs.

Bones

In order to understand the structure and function of the spine, we need to look more closely at how the components are arranged. The

5

Fig. 1: The Spine

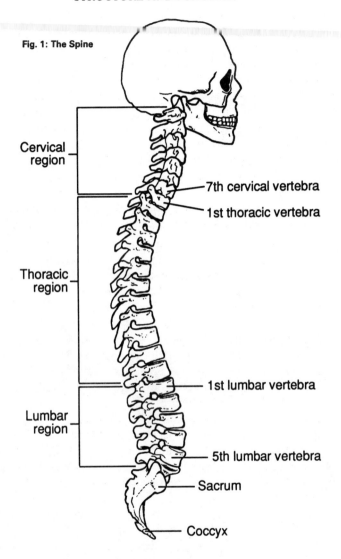

Cervical region

7th cervical vertebra

1st thoracic vertebra

Thoracic region

1st lumbar vertebra

Lumbar region

5th lumbar vertebra

Sacrum

Coccyx

vertebrae are stacked one on top of the other – like a pile of thick coins, but they do not form a straight vertical column. Viewed from the side, the spine has a series of gentle s-shaped curves. Thus the neck or cervical region has a curve that is convex forwards, the chest or thoracic region is convex backwards, and the back or lumbar region is again convex forwards; the sacrum is also curved, with its convexity backwards. This sinuous arrangement serves, among other things, to increase the shock-absorbing capacity of the spine.

No two vertebrae are exactly alike, but all are built on the same general plan (see Figure 2). Except in the upper two vertebrae (atlas and axis) there is a 'body', which is generally roundish and faces forwards. Behind this is a ring of bone called the neural arch. When the vertebrae are stacked on top of one another, as in life, the neural arches come together to form a tube, the spinal canal, which protects the important but vulnerable nerve, the spinal cord.

The vertebral arches are made up by the left and right 'little feet' (pedicles) that arise from the back of the vertebral body and by the thin blades (laminae) that close it behind. A vertebral spine projects backwards from each neural arch; in a fairly slim person these

Fig. 2: A Lumbar Vertebra

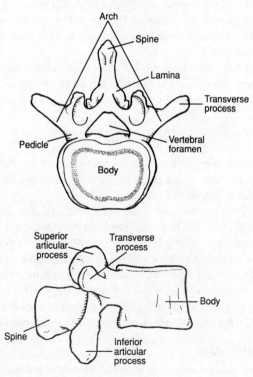

spines can easily be felt under the skin in the thoracic region. Other bony projections extend sideways from the arch and are called transverse processes, but they cannot be felt through the skin because they are covered by muscle. Still other pieces of bone, the four articular processes, project upwards and downwards from each vertebra and serve to link the vertebral column together.

The vertebrae are made of a type of bone called cancellous. This has a hard outer covering but inside it is filled with a network of bone like a sponge. Bones of this kind contain red marrow, which makes the red cells and some of the white cells of the blood.

We often think of bones as hard structures that do not change much in adult life. However, they are of course alive, and they are in fact capable of changing a great deal in certain circumstances, and quite rapidly too. If a bone is subjected to a load it tends to become stronger; conversely, if it is not loaded normally (for example, in someone ill in bed) it loses strength quickly. Pressure on a bone can cause it to change its shape in quite a short time, and so can an abnormal pull on a tendon or ligament that is attached to bone. For this reason someone suffering from a deformity of the spine (e.g. kyphosis or scoliosis) will acquire changes in the actual shape of his or her vertebrae.

The bones are covered by a special membrane called the periosteum. This helps to nourish the bone and plays a part in the repair process following a fracture.

Joints

Two kinds of joint are found in the spine. One is similar to the joints that exist in many other parts of the body, but the other is special and is found only in the spine.

Small facet joints unite each pair of articular processes (see Figure 3b). These are the same kind of synovial joint that is found in many other parts of the body, consisting of two opposed surfaces covered with a gristle-like cartilage substance – and surrounded by a protective capsule lined by a synovial membrane; they are lubricated by a special synovial fluid. Because the facet joints are of this kind they may be damaged by diseases, such as rheumatoid arthritis and osteoarthrosis, which affect synovial joints elsewhere.

Intervertebral discs

The other type of joint found in the vertebral column is unique to that situation. This the notorious intervertebral disc. Its function is to allow movement of the spine (bending forwards and backwards, together with some twisting) and also to provide shock absorption. Each disc consists of a ring of tough material – a substance called fibrous tissue – which is attached above and below to the adjacent vertebrae. The surfaces of the vertebral bodies facing the disc are covered with a thin end-plate of cartilage.

Fig. 3a: Intervertebral Disc (plan view)

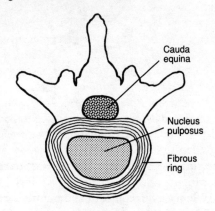

Fig. 3b: Intervertebral Discs (side view)

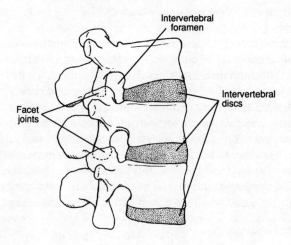

Fig. 3c: Cervical Spine (front view)

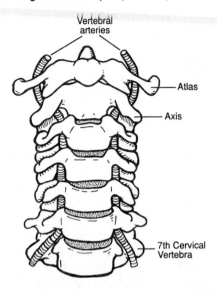

Inside the ring there is a jelly-like substance called the nucleus pulposus (see Figures 3a, b and c); it is this which provides the shock absorption. When a load is applied to the spine the nucleus pulposus is compressed, and because the fibrous ring is slightly elastic it bulges outwards, so allowing the vertebrae to come a little closer together. Because of our upright stance the spine is under continuous load all the time we are out of bed, and for this reason we are a little taller in the morning than in the evening. Indeed, astronauts, as they are not subjected to gravity, have been found to be as much as 10 cm taller on their return to earth.

The intervertebral discs are very firmly attached to the bones above and below and cannot 'slip' in the true sense. What happens in a so-called 'slipped disc' is that a crack develops in the fibrous ring, and this allows some or all of the nucleus pulposus to escape and press on surrounding structures, such as nerves.

The discs have very little blood supply. This means that healing of any damage will be slow, if it occurs at all. However, discs are not totally inert structures; they do need to be nourished and to receive oxygen, and for this they have to rely on the diffusion of fluid from the adjacent bones. This diffusion is assisted by the movements that occur naturally in the spine. Thus mobility helps maintain the health of the discs – one reason why exercise is important for the back.

Pelvic joints

The pelvis has rather unusual joints. The main ones are the two sacroiliac joints between the sacrum and the hip bones. These are synovial joints but they have very strong ligaments and rough surfaces, so that they move only a small amount. At the front of the pelvis the two hip bones meet in a joint called the symphysis pubis; again there is normally very little movement here.

Ligaments

These are tough bands or sheets of fibrous tissue that stretch between the bones and help to maintain the integrity of the spine. The character of the ligaments varies in the different regions of the spine. In the lower lumbar and pelvic regions they are particularly strong; in other areas they are more elastic, and one ligament, the so-called yellow ligament (ligamentum flavum), which connects the sides of the vertebral arches (the laminae) is particularly elastic. Like the intervertebral discs, the ligaments have a scanty blood supply and so are slow to heal when damaged.

Every joint in the body is supported by ligaments, which are important for stability and to limit movement. In most cases, however, the ligaments act as a kind of emergency brake on movement, most of the day-to-day control of the joints being supplied by muscles. But if a joint is subjected to too much strain, especially when the muscles are caught unawares, ligaments may be torn and the joint may even be dislocated, wholly or partially.

Muscles

The back contains some of the biggest and strongest muscles in the body. All are paired, and mostly they run alongside the spine, connecting varying numbers of vertebrae together or extending outwards into the limbs or ribs. The biggest and strongest muscles begin at the level of the pelvis and run up the spine for varying distances, being attached to the transverse processes and spines of the vertebrae, which act as levers for the muscles. Those in the chest are attached to the ribs and those in the neck to the skull.

An important pair of muscles that cannot be seen or felt from outside is the psoas muscles. These are inside the abdomen, where they are attached to the lumbar vertebrae, and they run down to the upper part of the thigh bone (femur). When the back is fixed they move the leg; when the leg is fixed they move the back.

Abdominal muscles

The abdominal muscles are also important for the back. These are mostly large sheets of muscle that are attached to the front of the pelvis and the lower ribs. When they contract they bend the spine forwards, and they also increase the pressure inside the abdomen; this helps to keep the spine from being injured during strong lifting. (It is for this reason that weight lifters wear a belt; and you have probably noticed that, when you lift a heavy weight, you automatically take a deep breath and hold it so as to give your abdominal muscles something to contract against.) People with slack abdominal muscles and 'pot bellies' are at increased risk of back pain and injury.

All these muscles are collectively responsible both for movement – bending and twisting – and for posture. Our ability to stand erect depends critically on the proper maintenance of the correct amount of tension in the various muscle groups. Even at rest, a muscle always preserves a certain degree of tension, which is called its tone.

Muscle tone

The tone of the muscles is maintained by a remarkable servo mechanism. Miniature structures in the muscles, called muscle spindles, constantly monitor the tension in the muscle. The muscle spindles are themselves little muscle fibres, with their own special motor as well as sensory nerve supply, so they can be 'set' by the central nervous system to adjust the tone of the main muscle as required. The muscle tone is also monitored by sense organs in the tendons.

Our ability to stand erect depends on muscle tone. If there were no muscles the spine would not keep upright but would droop. The spine is held up by the various muscles which keep adjusting their relative pulls – like the guy ropes of a tent. This does not require much effort, since once we are erect only slight adjustments are necessary. Naturally when we walk or run, or even if we move our arms, hundreds of complicated adjustments have to be made; all this is taken care of by the computing mechanisms in the spinal cord and cerebellum of the brain.

Nerves

The spinal cord

The spine encases and protects the spinal cord. The spinal cord is really an extension of the brain, and, like the brain, it contains nerve cells (neurones). The nerve cells control muscles and transmit sensation upwards to the brain. Together, the brain and spinal cord constitute the central nervous system; this is in contrast to the peripheral nervous system which is made up of the nerves that run out into the rest of the body.

Neither the brain nor its extension, the spinal cord, can regenerate if they are damaged. Sometimes other parts of the central nervous system can take over from the damaged area and replace some of its functions, but the damaged cells themselves do not recover. This is in contrast to what happens in the peripheral nervous system, where damaged nerves can regrow and restore function to the parts of the body they supply.

The spinal cord extends from the base of the skull to the junction of the first and second lumbar vertebrae. However, the sheath around it (dura mater) extends as far as the sacrum, and this allows doctors to take samples of the fluid surrounding the cord without damaging the cord itself.

The way in which the nerves arise from the spinal cord is important. The cord is arranged segmentally (this is a relic from our ancestry; segmental arrangements of nerves can be found in many kinds of animals, even earthworms) (see Figure 4).

A series of left and right nerve root pairs emerges from the cord. On each side the nerve roots are double, one in front and one

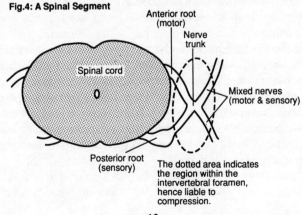

Fig.4: A Spinal Segment

Anterior root (motor)

Nerve trunk

Spinal cord

Mixed nerves (motor & sensory)

Posterior root (sensory)

The dotted area indicates the region within the intervertebral foramen, hence liable to compression.

13

behind. The front (ventral) root is mainly motor (concerned with muscles and movement) and the rear (dorsal) root is sensory (bringing sense impulses from the skin and other structures to the spinal cord and, ultimately, the brain). The two roots unite to form a nerve trunk, and this in turn branches to give rise to the various nerves that run to the different parts of the body. Since these nerves are made up of a mixture of fibres from the two nerve roots, they carry both motor and sensory impulses.

The nerve trunks emerge from the spine through gaps between the vertebrae. These gaps are called the intervertebral foramina [sing. foramen]. The roots carry with them a prolongation of the dura mater that covers the spinal cord. Because the spinal cord ends at the bottom of the first lumbar vertebrae, the nerve roots that leave by the foramina below this level have quite a long way to go to reach their destination; hence in this region of the spine there is a sheaf of nerve roots, which is called the horse's tail (the cauda equina).

The way in which the nerve roots are arranged means that they are liable to be squeezed if the intervertebral foramen becomes narrowed for any reason: for example, if a disc collapses, bringing two vertebrae closer together, or if a facet joint becomes diseased and swollen. Many of the symptoms of back pain are due to nerve root compression arising at this site.

The segmental arrangement of the spinal nerve roots has important consequences for diagnosis. The different spinal segments have a pretty constant relationship to the various parts of the body. Thus, weakness and wasting of the small muscles of the hand points to some form of damage at the level of the lower cervical or upper thoracic segments, while pain in the big toe due to nerve root compression must be coming from the lower lumbar or upper sacral nerve roots.

In addition to the motor and sensory nervous system there is also what is called the autonomic nervous system. This controls activities such as heart rate, glandular function, movements of the intestine, and contraction and dilatation of the pupils – activities that are not under voluntary control. It is customary to subdivide the autonomic nervous system into a sympathetic and a parasympathetic part: the sympathetic system is broadly responsible for responses to emergencies (fright and flight) while the parasympathetic system tends to maintain the automatic processes on which we rely during the course of our ordinary activities; however, this division is not

14

absolute. The actions of sympathetic and parasympathetic systems often oppose each other, the outcome being a constantly shifting balance; our heart rate, for example, is determined by the interaction between the two systems, which is why the rate increases when we are anxious (the balance shifts towards the sympathetic pole).

Blood vessels

Like other structures, the back is critically dependent on its blood supply. Arteries and veins supply the bones, nerves, and muscles, and interference with the blood supply for any reason will cause damage.

In the cervical region the spine affords passage for a particularly important pair of blood vessels, called the vertebral arteries. These pass up through special openings in the transverse processes on each side; at the top of the spine the left and right vertebral arteries unite to form the basilar artery, which supplies the brain-stem. In elderly patients disease of the cervical portion of the spine can compress the vertebral arteries, so that looking upwards or turning the head can cause giddiness or sudden unconsciousness. (The stem is the part of the brain most closely concerned with the maintenance of consciousness.)

Connective tissue

Although often forgotten, the connective tissue is an important component of the back. It is a kind of 'packing' tissue that surrounds the various organs and structures in the body; if all the other material were removed, the connective tissue would remain as a kind of ghost, outlining the form of the body. It is largely made up of a substance called collagen but it also contains a number of different kinds of cells.

Attachments of other structures

The head
The skull is joined to the rest of the spine by two special vertebrae. The uppermost of these is the atlas, which is named after the legendary giant in Greek mythology who carried the world on his

15

shoulders. The atlas is an approximately circular vertebra which lacks a true body; it has upward-facing facet joints that allow the head to make nodding movements (see Fig. 5).

Fig. 5: Skull and Neck

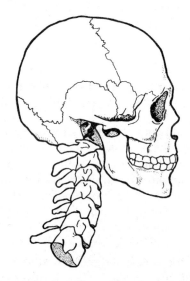

Immediately below the atlas is the axis. This provides for rotation (twisting) movements. The considerable weight of the head is kept in place by a special peg of bone (the odontoid process) that projects upwards from the axis to prevent the atlas and skull from sliding about. If the odontoid process is broken, as can happen in a severe whiplash injury, the atlas may slip and break the upper part of the spinal cord, causing immediate death.

The arms

Our upper arms are attached quite loosely to the spine, by muscles and connective tissue rather than actual joints. The upper arm bone (humerus) is fixed to the shoulder blade (scapula) by a very shallow 'ball-and-socket' joint. But the scapula itself is not connected directly to the spine; instead, it slides over the chest wall, to which it is linked by muscles. The only direct connection between limb and trunk is that between the collar bone (clavicle) and the breast bone (sternum). This arrangement allows maximum freedom of movement for the arms, at the cost of some reduction in strength.

16

The ribs

There are 12 pairs of ribs, each of which is attached at the back to a thoracic vertebra. The ribs move a fair amount on the spine, so as to permit the chest to expand in breathing.

Very occasionally people have an extra rib on one or both sides of their neck, attached to the seventh cervical vertebra. This may cause symptoms by pressing on nerves or blood vessels, although it does not necessarily do so.

The legs

In contrast to the arms, the legs have very strong attachments to the spine via the pelvis, which is made up of the sacrum and the left and right hip bones. The hip joints are deep ball-and-socket joints, which are reinforced by strong ligaments. Other ligaments connect the sacrum and hip bones and also the lower lumbar vertebrae and the hip bones, so that the whole structure is almost rigid. There is some movement between the various bones of the pelvis but not very much.

Anatomical variations

Anatomy textbooks describe the typical appearance of the spine and other structures in the body. However, no two people are exactly alike (apart from 'identical' twins), and sometimes x-rays or other tests show unexpected variations from the 'normal'. It is possible for some of these variations to cause symptoms: a cervical rib may press on structures, for example, or an abnormal lumbar vertebra may give rise to instability of the spine. However, it is by no means necessary for this to happen; many of us have anatomical peculiarities that we are happily unaware of, and even if symptoms do occur it is often difficult to be sure that they are caused by any abnormalities that may be present.

Differences among the various regions

There are numerous structural differences among the various regions of the back.

The cervical or neck region is the most mobile and the most lightly built. Movements can occur quite freely in all planes (fore and aft, side to side, and rotation), and fine control is provided by numerous muscles including some small ones at the base of the skull. Many important arteries, veins and nerves, as well as the windpipe (trachea) and gullet (oesophagus) traverse the region.

The thoracic or chest region is less mobile, and indeed in middle-aged and elderly patients it may be almost fixed. The main movements are in the fore and aft plane, although there is also some rotation.

The lumbar or back region is solidly built. Some fore and aft movement is permitted but little rotation.

The pelvis is almost completely rigid, although a little nodding movement occurs at the sacroiliac joints. Note that the pelvis is angled so that its opening faces slightly forwards as well as upwards.

Function of the back as a whole

Although it is convenient to divide the spine into sections for purposes of description, it is important to realize that the back functions as a whole unit. If we turn our head, for example, it is not only the muscles of the neck that have to cooperate; small readjustments of tone must occur in all the muscles of the back in order to preserve our posture. Large-scale movements such as walking or running involve many hundreds of muscles, which are controlled by an incredibly complex computer program that we ordinarily take for granted – until something goes wrong. This coordination is carried out below the level of consciousness by the nervous system. The mechanisms responsible exist mainly in the spinal cord and in the structure at the base of the brain called the cerebellum.

2
What Goes Wrong

It is often difficult to give patients an exact answer when they ask what is wrong with their backs. This is partly because, at least until recently, it has not been possible to investigate the mechanism of the living back in any great detail. Today, thanks to modern methods of imaging such as CT and MRI scanning (see p. 53), things are beginning to change, but even so a full explanation of a patient's pain is often not forthcoming, owing to the sheer complexity of the back. In many cases more than one mechanism of pain production is involved.

Some back disorders are due to specific diseases, but many others are simply the result of the ageing process. 'Ageing' in this sense begins quite early: changes are discernible even in our twenties, although symptoms seldom arise until a decade or two later.

The Ageing Back and Spondylosis

There is often confusion in people's minds about the terms used to describe the changes that occur with age.

'Is it arthritis?'

People are sometimes told that they are suffering from 'arthritis of the spine'. This diagnosis can cause a good deal of alarm: patients may assume that they have a progressive disease that will eventually confine them to a wheelchair. Fortunately, this is not generally the case.

There are two common kinds of arthritis: rheumatoid arthritis, which is a generalized disease affecting many joints as well as other organs and tissues, and osteoarthritis (osteoarthrosis). It is generally osteoarthritis that affects the spine in older people.

The cause of this disorder is not clearly understood. It may take various forms. Sometimes it affects just one or two joints, especially large weight-bearing joints such as the knee or the hip. At other times, particularly in middle-aged women, it affects mainly the hands, where it causes swelling and deformity of the joints nearest to the finger tips. (Rheumatoid arthritis, in contrast, typically causes swelling and deformity of the wrists and knuckles.)

19

Osteoarthritis certainly can affect the spine, but some of the changes that occur in the spine with age are not due to this disease but arise in other ways. These changes are known collectively as 'spondylosis', which is often described to the patient as 'wear and tear'. It is better to use this term rather than 'arthritis', because what is being described is less a disease than the more or less inevitable deterioration that accompanies ageing. Osteoarthritis may well be present in addition, but applying the term as a label may give patients an unduly gloomy impression of their prospects.

Even the description 'wear and tear' may be too pessimistic, with its implication that time is passing and nothing can be done. Although it is true that most people of middle age or older will show the changes referred to as spondylosis to a greater or lesser degree, this does not necessarily mean that they must suffer a proportionate amount of pain. Indeed, they may well have no symptoms at all.

There is in any case only an approximate correlation between the degree of degenerative change that may be present and the patient's age. In some people these changes begin much earlier than in others. This is partly a matter of heredity – susceptibility to 'wear-and-tear' can run in families – but it can also be related to occupation: heavy labouring may cause early degenerative changes in the spine, and so can certain sports or recreations. Professional footballers quite often suffer from osteoarthritis of the knees later in life, and gymnasts who enter competition when they are too young may pay for it later in terms of their spines.

The main features of spondylosis

Spondylosis appears in two main sites: the facet joints and the discs.

The facet joints The facet joints of the spine, being synovial joints like, for example, the knee or the wrist, are liable to the same kinds of disease as those that affect synovial joints elsewhere in the body. Osteoarthrosis of these joints may give rise to pain directly, or it may cause the joints to swell and so narrow the intervertebral foramina; this in turn may cause pressure on nerve roots, giving rise to secondary (referred) pain.

The role of these small joints in the production of back pain is sometimes forgotten; people tend to place undue emphasis on the more fashionable discs. However the facet joints are very important in this respect.

20

The intervertebral discs Like the facet joints, these tend to deteriorate with age. The patient may never have suffered an episode of acute backache, but an x-ray may show that one or more of the intervertebral discs is thinner than normal. This thinning indicates that the soft part of the discs concerned (the nucleus pulposus) has escaped at some time. Even if this jelly material has not pressed on any nerve roots, the resulting loss of disc space may cause narrowing of the intervertebral foramina and so compress the nerve roots. This compression may be increased if there is also swelling of the facet joints, as there may well be.

The notorious 'slipped disc' really refers to escape (prolapse) of disc contents (see p. 10). It is usually the final stage in a process of gradual weakening of the disc. It may occur at any level in the spine, although most commonly in the lumbar region, where it can give rise to sciatica. Sometimes more than one disc is involved.

Disc prolapse may occur in any direction. If the material moves forwards there may be few or no symptoms, but if it moves backwards it is liable to press on nerve roots or on the spinal cord. Most frequently the disc material goes back and to one or other side, which explains the common occurrence of one-sided sciatica. It is also possible for disc material to escape into the body of the vertebrae through cracks in the cartilaginous end-plate; this gives rise to pain in the back although not to pressure on nerves. In some cases the disc merely bulges, without actually rupturing; in such cases there may be only back pain, without associated nerve root symptoms. When nerve root symptoms do occur they constitute a form of referred pain (see pp. 22–3).

Other changes Other features of age-related degeneration may be evident on x-ray. The most dramatic of these is often the appearance of osteophytes: outgrowths of bony tissue; these are typically seen at the margins of the vertebral bodies. Although they may appear impressive, osteophytes frequently give rise to no symptoms, unless they happen to occur in an area where they compress nerve tissue. Quite often they merely limit the movement of the spine without causing any pain; it is possible that in such cases they are actually providing a degree of protection for the spine.

A different kind of change, which is almost the opposite of that just described, consists of the development of instability of the spinal joints. Vertebrae may slip or move on one another (spondylolisthesis). Sometimes this is a consequence of degenerative weakness, or it may be a congenital abnormality. It is yet another cause of nerve root compression.

The various regions of the back tend to be affected by these changes in different ways and to different extents. The most significant effects are usually seen in the cervical and lumbar regions. The neck is vulnerable because it is the most mobile part of the spine, whereas the lumbar region suffers because it carries so much of the body weight. Disease in either of these areas can cause the spine to lose its normal curvature, or alternatively can increase the curvature to an abnormal extent, giving rise to deformity – kyphosis and scoliosis (see p. 27).

Pain in spondylosis

There are a number of ways in which spondylosis can give rise to back pain. Osteoarthrosis itself may be painful. Instability of the joints of the back or excessive lordosis can place undue strain on the ligaments, which then become painful. Sometimes, when the disc space has been lost, the bones may come together and press on each other ('kissing spines').

The commonest cause of spondolytic pain, however, is probably compression of nerves or nerve roots. The cause is often, though certainly not invariably, prolapse of a disc ('slipped disc'). The characteristic symptom of such compression is referred pain. This is pain which is felt, not in the area which is damaged, but some distance away.

In the case of nerve root compression this is perhaps not very difficult to understand. It is rather as if a central office were to receive incoming fax messages that had been generated, not in an outlying office, but by some interference with the telephone lines; this might lead the central office to think that its subsidiary was experiencing problems which were, in fact, being generated elsewhere.

There are other kinds of referred pain which are harder to understand, and which seem to depend on alterations in the way in which patterns of messages are processed by the central nervous system. This may explain some of the bizarre sensations, such as feelings of heat and cold, or of running water, that some patients with back disorders report.

In the neck, nerve root pressure may give rise to pain in the arms, which may reach down as far as the hands. In the lumbar (back) region nerve root pressure can give rise to pain in the buttocks, thighs, calves or feet – sciatica. (Pain in the lower limbs is often called sciatica even when, as may be the case, the nerve affected is not in fact the sciatic but another nerve which originates in the lumbar region, such as the femoral nerve.)

Narrowing of the spinal canal in the neck or (less commonly) the thorax may compress the spinal cord in these regions, giving rise to symptoms of weakness in the legs because long nerve fibres from the brain traverse the cord in these regions on their way to the legs. (This is the reason why doctors test the reflexes in the legs when examining a patient with symptoms of neck disease.) Disease of the lumbar spine can also cause weakness of the legs, but it is of a different type because the spinal cord does not reach this far down.

Muscle spasm In many cases of back pain, especially those which have come on acutely, there is a greater or lesser degree of muscle spasm. Sometimes the spasm is so severe that the back cannot move at all; in other cases the patient may not even be aware of it. The spasm serves a purpose: it splints the spine and preserves it from further injury, but it is often said that the muscles that are in spasm are painful. Whether this is actually true, however, is difficult to establish; muscle spasm is not always painful, and it is possible that when pain is present in such cases it is produced in other ways. Muscle spasm relaxes as the underlying injury heals.

Trigger points An increasing number of doctors today recognize the existence of another source of pain in the back (and elsewhere). Many patients have zones in their muscles, and sometimes in other tissues as well, such as ligaments, which hurt when pressed. The muscles may also feel more tense than normal; sometimes this takes the form of taut bands in the muscles. These are known as 'trigger points'.

Almost everyone has a few of these, and indeed in some places they could be regarded as normal; for example, in the centre of the trapezius muscle on top of the shoulder. In some people, however, the trigger points become unduly sensitive, so that they may be painful when pressed quite lightly or even without being touched at all. They may then cause pain to radiate to other areas; that is, they are a source of referred pain.

Not much is known about what trigger points really are or how they arise. They have, in fact, largely been ignored by mainstream medicine, although they have been described under other names in the past: fibrositis or muscular rheumatism, for example. Attempts have been made to find out what they are by removing them surgically for examination under a microscope (taking a biopsy), but on inspection few changes have been found. Possibly, trigger points are simply the result of localized increases in blood flow; this would fit in with the observation that they can come and go very quickly, in response to pressure or other things.

Trigger points are important because they can give rise to many of the symptoms that are generally thought to be due to nerve root compression. They may, for example, cause sciatica or pain in the arms and hands. It seems likely that a good deal of back pain and its associated manifestations is in fact due mainly to the presence of these trigger points, instead of – or as well as – actual compression of nerves by disease of the bones and joints.

If the existence and importance of trigger points is recognized, then for many patients with back pain, considerable relief may be obtained because it is possible to treat them in various ways, especially by acupuncture (see pp. 68–74).

Back pain from other causes

In addition to the mainly 'wear-and-tear' changes described so far, there are a number of other possible causes for back pain. I want to emphasize that *most are rare*. By far the most common causes of back pain are the kinds of disorder discussed already – i.e., mechanical problems affecting the joints or muscles. The remaining disease categories (which will seem daunting) are mentioned for the sake of completeness. Unfortunately, it is not possible to provide a checklist of symptoms that will allow you to decide for yourself what kind of back pain you are suffering from. The only safe advice that can be given is that if you are suffering from 'new' back pain that lasts more than a few days you ought to see your family doctor. This is particularly true if you are middle-aged or elderly.

Inflammation

In every-day language, 'inflammation' suggests the sort of appearance that occurs when a wound becomes infected. The classic signs of inflammation are pain, redness, heat and swelling. Under the microscope certain characteristic changes can be seen, such as an increase in blood flow and in the number of white blood cells in the affected tissues.

Inflammation of the spinal joints is characterized by microscopic changes of this kind, and pain occurs too; however, swelling, although present, is not apparent from the outside owing to the thickness of the muscles overlying the spine.

Rheumatoid arthritis

Rheumatoid arthritis is an inflammatory disease of the joints, and can affect the spine, although it is usually less prominent here than elsewhere in the body. It gives rise to stiffness and loss of mobility; occasionally it can cause a dangerous instability of the joint between the atlas and the axis (see p. 7). Although fortunately rare, this is a complication requiring urgent treatment by a specialist.

Ankylosing spondylitis

Ankylosing spondylitis, in contrast, does affect, typically the spine. It is commoner in men than in women and there is a tendency for the disease to run in families. It causes stiffness as well as pain, and in severe cases the spine may become totally rigid. Fortunately, however, many patients have only mild symptoms. Anti-inflammatory drugs can help to control the symptoms, and sufferers are encouraged to keep as mobile as possible.

Reiter's disease

Reiter's disease is an inflammation of the spine that may (rarely) follow an attack of urethritis. Other joints, such as the knees, are often involved as well.

Osteoporosis

This condition is the result of the progressive loss of the body's calcium stores. It affects everyone as they get older to some extent but is particularly troublesome for women after the menopause. The loss of calcium does not in itself usually cause symptoms, but the bones become weaker and more likely to break with even minor stresses. In the spine this weakness causes the bodies of the vertebrae to collapse, and this gives rise to pain locally. If nerve roots are pressed on by the collapsed vertebrae there will be referred pain and other distant effects. As more vertebrae collapse the person tends to lose height, and osteoporotic collapse is one cause of the 'dowager's hump' that afflicts some elderly women. There may also be pain from the bones even in the absence of

25

vertebral collapse; one theory is that this is caused by distension of the veins within the vertebrae.

It is difficult to help osteoporosis once it has occurred. However, the rate at which calcium is lost from the skeleton can be reduced in various ways. Exercise helps to preserve the strength of the bones. In women, oestrogen given as hormone replacement therapy after the menopause also slows bone loss and can probably even reverse it. Small thin women are particularly at risk of developing osteoporosis, as are those whose ovaries have been removed before their natural menopause.

It is undoubtedly important for children and adolescents to have a good calcium intake in order to build up an adequate reserve of bone, but whether calcium supplements are helpful in later life is uncertain. To take excessive amounts of calcium and vitamin D is certainly unwise and may give rise to kidney stones. Vitamin D deficiency does not cause osteoporosis, but does cause a different disorder characterized by softening of the bones; in adults this is called osteomalacia; in children rickets.

Vertebral fracture

Even in the absence of osteoporosis, vertebrae may of course be broken like any other bones. A fall from a height, especially landing on the buttocks, can jar the spine and cause a vertebral body to collapse. Other fractures can affect the vertebral arch or separate the arch from the body of the vertebra (spondylolysis). A very strong contraction of a back muscle may occasionally break off one of the transverse processes to which the muscle is attached.

There is generally no specific treatment for these fractures; patients are given pain-relieving drugs and the fracture is allowed to mend by itself. A major exception to this is a fracture of the odontoid process of the axis, below the skull; for reasons already explained (see p. 25) this is an emergency and requires urgent attention from a surgeon.

Injury to the coccyx can give rise to severe pain. Some people – usually women – suffer severe pain in the region of the coccyx even without having suffered an injury; the cause of this pain is often obscure, and it can be difficult to relieve.

As well as fractures, accidental injuries can cause other kinds of damage to the spine. Particularly in the neck and upper back regions the thin plate of cartilage adjacent to a disc may crack, allowing disc material to escape into the vertebral body; there may also be a disc prolapse (see p. 21).

Scoliosis

Scoliosis refers to an abnormal twisting and sideways bending deformity of the spine. It can occur in various ways. When there is acute back pain for any reason the muscles of the spine may go into spasm in order to limit movement and prevent further damage. If the degree of spasm on the two sides of the back is unequal, as it may be, scoliosis will result, but this is temporary and disappears as the patient recovers.

A different type of scoliosis (idiopathic scoliosis) sometimes occurs for unknown reasons in adolescent girls. At first it is slight, but the disorder tends to worsen as the girl grows and eventually it may become severe. Sometimes surgery is necessary to correct the deformity.

Scheuermann's disease (vertebral osteochondrosis)

Like idiopathic scoliosis, this disorder usually occurs in the growing spine and affects mainly teenagers. It is thought to be due to the nuclear pulp protruding into a vertebral body through a defect. It may cause little disturbance, or it may lead to severe disturbance of growth and cause kyphosis – a form of 'hunchback'.

Arachnoiditis

The arachnoid membrane is one of the three coverings of the brain and spinal cord. The termination '-itis' means 'inflammation', so arachnoiditis is inflammation of the arachnoid membrane. At one time it was sometimes seen after an oil-based insoluble fluid had been injected into the spine in order to show it up on x-rays, but this no longer occurs because the modern dyes are water-based. However, arachnoiditis still occurs at times, sometimes after operations on the back. It can also occur after various infections or for unknown reasons. It does not always cause symptoms but it can give rise to persistent pain which at present is difficult to treat. Sometimes it clears up spontaneously without treatment.

Paget's disease

This is a disorder of bone whose cause is unknown; one theory is that it is due to a virus. Areas of bone are destroyed, following which repair occurs. It may affect any of the bones, including the vertebrae, but is particularly common in the lumbar spine and the pelvis. The skull may also be affected. There may be no symptoms at all, or it may give rise to persistent pain. There is no cure at present; pain-relieving drugs are used as necessary.

Cancer

Although this is by no means a common cause of back pain, the doctor always has to keep the possibility in mind when seeing a middle-aged or elderly patient with symptoms that have come on fairly recently. Tumours of various organs, but especially the breast in women and the prostate in men, may cause deposits of cancer cells in the bones of the spine. Tumours may also arise in the spine itself, although these are rare.

Pain in the spine caused by cancer may be treated by x-rays, which usually give good relief.

Migraine

Migraine usually causes headaches. However, very occasionally people suffer from migraine-like symptoms in other parts of the body, including the back. In such cases episodes of pain occur for no apparent reason at intervals of weeks or months. This is such an unusual cause for back pain that an opinion from a neurologist is generally required before it can be made with any confidence, but it is worth considering in cases where no other explanation can be found.

Gout

This is a disease caused by a high level of uric acid in the blood. We usually think of gout as affecting the big toe, but other joints, including those of the spine, may be involved. Patients may experience severe backache at the same time as pain in their toes or other peripheral joints, and there may be severe pain in the muscles of the back, so that it is almost impossible to move. Gouty patients seem to be particularly liable to suffer painful osteoarthritis of the spine.

Polymyalgia rheumatica

This is an important if not very common cause of pain in the shoulder or hip girdles. It is important partly because it is very easily treated once diagnosed but also because it may be associated with temporal arteritis, which can cause blindness if untreated.

28

Polymyalgia rheumatica affects women much more than men and usually occurs after the age of 60. It can come on very suddenly and is characterized by severe muscle pain. Treatment is by corticosteroids, which keep it under control until it clears up spontaneously, which it usually does after some months or years.

Tuberculosis

In former times tuberculosis was an important cause of spinal disease, especially in children, but it has now become very rare; however, with the decline in vaccination against tuberculosis it is possible that it will begin to reappear. Patients used to have to spend months or years encased in plaster casts, unable to move, but modern anti-tubercle drugs control the disease in a much shorter time.

Pain referred to the back from elsewhere

Just as disease in the spine can cause referred pain in other areas, so disease of various organs can cause referred pain in the back. This is particularly the case in women; a prolapsed uterus, for example, can cause low back pain. Another example is disease of a kidney, such as a kidney stone, which can give rise to back pain.

In the past, back pain due to disease of various organs, especially the womb, was over-diagnosed; many women had hysterectomies to remove their wombs or operations to correct the position of the womb which were unnecessary. Pain referred to the back from internal organs certainly does occur, but perhaps not as commonly as used to be thought.

3

The Characteristics of Back Pain

Types of pain

In broad terms there are three kinds of spinal pain:

1. pain arising from the 'motion segment';
2. pain affecting the superficial tissues;
3. pain occuring when a spinal nerve is compressed.

This neat division of pain into three types is convenient, but in practice it is often difficult to decide where the site of a patient's trouble lies. This is because the three kinds often occur together.

The first kind of spinal pain arises from the 'motion segment'; that is, a pair of vertebrae and the joints between them, consisting of the intervertebral disc and the two facet joints, as well as the muscles and ligaments in that region. Any of these structures can give rise to pain. There are 23 motion segments in all.

Pain arising from a motion segment has a deep, dull aching quality, and it may radiate to other areas in a way that is difficult to explain in terms of the known nervous system. For example, pain from the cervical spine may radiate to the eye, chest wall and elbow; pain in the thoracic spine may be felt in the front of the body, giving rise to a mistaken diagnosis of abdominal pain; and in the lumbar region there may be radiation to the groin, lower abdomen and foot. Changes in blood flow in these regions can occur, and patients may experience sweating or nausea. Pain is often referred from various motion segments to the sacroiliac joint (see p. 11), and this joint then becomes tender although it is not itself the site of trouble. (Pain from the sacroiliac joint is felt in the buttock and down the leg.)

The second type of spinal pain affects the superficial tissues, including the skin, the superficial ligaments and muscles, and the tips of the spinous processes of the vertebrae. This kind of pain can be accurately localized to the site of trouble. An example is the pain caused by 'kissing spines'; this is felt when the back is straight but disappears when the patient bends forward.

The third type of pain occurs when a spinal nerve is compressed as it emerges through an intervertebral foramen. This kind of pain is sharp and 'electric' in character; it can be intense. It is similar to the sensation felt on hitting the 'funny bone' (ulnar nerve) in the elbow. There is often impairment of sensation or increase in sensitivity to touch in the area of skin supplied by the affected nerve, and this helps the doctor to identify the spinal segment involved. If the motor function of the nerve is affected there may be weakness and ultimately wasting of the muscles supplied by the nerve, and the limb reflexes, such as the knee jerk, may be lost.

There are wide variations in what makes the pain better or worse. Some people feel worse standing, others feel worse sitting or even lying down. Coughing and sneezing may also make the pain worse. Bending may be all but impossible, or the back may move quite freely. The back itself may be very sensitive to pressure, sometimes just over one or two vertebrae, or there may be no tenderness at all.

Back pain is often worse at night – perhaps partly because there are fewer distractions to take the patient's mind off the pain at this time. Lying down usually relieves stresses on joints but not always; sometimes it makes matters worse. Most patients with osteoarthritis find that they stiffen up with prolonged rest and this may be another aggravating factor. Changes in position during sleep may also play a part. However, if pain is always worse at night, regardless of the position one lies in, this is unusual and requires further investigation.

Quality of pain

The quality of pain is notoriously difficult to describe. Patients may say their pain is throbbing, which indicates a beating or pounding sensation in time with the pulse. When present it suggests inflammation from some cause. 'Shooting' pains may occur in sciatica, either spontaneously or in response to particular movements. Some patients experience a 'catch' as a joint moves through a particular part of its range. A common complaint is of 'burning' pain when certain postures are adopted, especially with the neck.

Role of the autonomic nervous system

Although most of the referred-pain symptoms described so far are attributable to damage to the ordinary sensory nerves, the body contains another nervous system, called the autonomic nervous system (see pp. 14–15). This may also be involved in back disorders. Patients may complain of pallor or flushing, hearing disorders and tinnitus, decreased visual acuity, alterations of sensation in the face or scalp, and a feeling of a lump in the throat. Such symptoms may in part be due to autonomic disturbance. Probably pain can also be transmitted by the autonomic nervous system. The multiplicity of symptoms that can be caused in this way may make doctors suspect that a patient's symptoms are psychological, but this is often a mistake.

Patterns of onset of pain

It is customary to classify symptoms and disorders depending on how they occur, into three groups. *Acute* means a fairly sudden onset – generally within 24 hours – in a person who was previously in good health from that point of view. (Sometimes a subdivision called *subacute* is used to signify a more gradual onset, perhaps lasting a few days, but again in someone who was previously healthy.) Someone whose back suddenly 'locks' so that he cannot move has experienced acute pain. Notice, incidentally, that this use of the word is not quite the same as the popular usage; in medical terminology to say that a pain is acute does not necessarily imply that it is very severe, although of course it often is.

Recurrent symptoms are those that keep going away and coming back at intervals of months or even years. Many instances of back pain come into this category. The recurrences may or may not be precipitated by an obvious cause.

Chronic pain is long-lasting. Once again, the word does not say anything about the severity of the pain, only about its duration. Chronic back pain may come on insidiously, it may follow a number of recurrent episodes, or it may stem from an acute episode from which the patient fails to recover. There is no fixed time limit after which an episode of back pain would be said to have become chronic, although if there has been no recovery or an incomplete one after three months most doctors would probably say that the disorder has entered the chronic stage.

Symptom patterns in different areas

Each region of the back tends to have its own characteristic types of pain.

The neck region (cervical spine)

Acute torticollis (wry neck)

This tends to afflict young people particularly. The patient wakes up one morning to find that his or her neck is painful and cannot be turned far in one or other direction. With or without treatment, recovery usually occurs within a few days, although it may take ten days or more.

The cause of this illness is unknown. Some people move surprisingly vigorously when asleep, twisting, turning, kicking, grinding their teeth and so on, so it is possible that they contort their necks into an unnatural position and strain the muscles or joints. The opposite can also occur: during dreaming sleep the muscles are profoundly relaxed, so that the neck may fall into an unnatural posture and this, too, can strain the joints. Either of these mechanisms could slightly displace (subluxate) one of the facet joints in the neck, or it could cause a disc to bulge slightly owing to a slow shift of disc substance during sleep.

Although complete recovery is the rule, the duration of the pain can often be reduced by treatment by physical means (acupuncture or osteopathy).

Cervical spondylosis

In older patients, the commonest cause of neck pain is cervical spondylosis. But it is vital to understand that the mere presence of wear-and-tear changes on x-ray does not in itself account for a patient's symptoms. Even x-ray evidence that a particular inter-vertebral foramen has been narrowed does not necessarily prove that the patient's symptoms are due to this. Nevertheless, it is important not to go too far in the opposite direction: cervical spondylosis can certainly give rise to symptoms in its own right.

In addition to the joints of the neck, the muscles of the neck and their associated trigger points can also be an important source of symptoms. The neck muscles have an extraordinarily hard task to perform. To get an idea of the amount of work they have to do, take an 8 lb (4 kg) weight in your hand to represent the head, and with your elbow resting on a table hold the weight vertically. Now try moving the weight about by bending your wrist, and you will begin to appreciate the strain that the joints and muscles of the neck have to cope with during the day. It is hardly surprising that, after forty or fifty years of this, they may begin to protest a little. It is also not surprising that there can be many mechanisms involved in the production of symptoms in this region of the body.

Symptoms can occur in many ways. They may be present mainly in the morning, as a result of strains experienced during sleep, or they may come on during the course of habitual day time activities, such as driving or working at a desk. Symptoms may be precipitated by fairly minor stresses: painting a ceiling, a dog pulling on a lead, or an unusually long period of reading or sewing. Typically, there is a vague pain in the neck at first, with some stiffness; later the pain spreads to the top of the shoulder (trapezius muscle) and the upper part of the arm. Usually the pain is one-sided, although both sides may be affected, and movement of the neck towards the painful side makes it worse.

The pain and stiffness may get better – partially or completely – after a few weeks or months, but it will often come back a few months later, sometimes more severely; later on it may disappear once more. Now, there may be tingling in the hands and weakness of some of the small muscles in the hands. Pain at this time often has a peculiar, 'toothachy' quality which makes it particularly unpleasant. There may be radiation of pain to the back of the head or to the forehead and eyes; patients often describe this as headache. Some people experience crawling sensations or feelings of heat in the scalp.

The normal appearance of the neck may alter, giving rise to a 'dowager's hump' at the base of the neck. The muscles and tissues beneath the skin may become thickened and stiff.

Older patients may complain of dizziness (vertigo) as well as pain; sometimes dizziness is the only symptom. The cause is often said to be pressure on the vertebral arteries (see p. 15), but in many cases the explanation is probably disease of the facet joints affecting the balance mechanism.

We maintain our balance by a constant delicate readjustment of muscle tone, and the complex computing system responsible for this relies on information about our position from a number of sources: our eyes, the balance organs in our inner ears, and the special sense organs in our muscles and joints that tell us the position of our limbs even when we are not looking at them. The facet joints in the neck are particularly important in this respect. They supply information about the position of the head in relation to the trunk, and this is vital for the maintenance of balance. When these joints are distorted by osteoarthrosis they may produce abnormal messages that confuse the brain and interfere with its balance control.

Pain may be referred to the back of the head, owing to compression of the nerves that arise in the neck and supply that area. If the spinal cord is compressed by narrowing in the spinal canal at the neck there may be weakness of the legs and the gait may be affected.

Whiplash injury

A common cause of neck problems these days is whiplash injury. If a vehicle is struck from behind in a traffic accident the passengers are thrown violently forwards. Their heads, however, tend to lag behind the movement of their trunks, and so their necks are bent strongly backwards, straining the joints and ligaments. In the immediate aftermath this causes pain in the neck and sometimes tingling in the arms and hands. There may also be pain in the face or throat, a feeling of numbness of the face, pain in the ears or the eyes, disturbances of hearing or vision, a need to keep clearing the throat compulsively, giddiness, fatigue and depression, irritability, and inability to sleep.

In past years doctors have often suspected that many of these symptoms are psychological or even connected with a desire to obtain a good compensation settlement after a road traffic accident. However, recent research suggests that this is seldom the case; most patients do have a physical cause for their symptoms and these do not usually disappear even after the question of compensation has been settled.

Symptoms may continue for months or even years, even though x-rays of the neck show no abnormality; this seems to happen particularly in women. The cause is uncertain, although many patients have persisting muscle trigger points, and treatment of these can be helpful.

Prevention is important: head restraints should be fitted to car seats and should reach high enough to stop the head from moving backwards. Restraints that reach only to the back of the neck or the base of the skull are worse than useless, since they merely provide a pivot round which the neck can rotate and stretch even further than it otherwise would.

Neck tension

Probably the commonest cause of pain in the neck is neck tension. The patient (usually a woman of middle age or younger) complains of chronic aching in the neck, usually mainly on one side. The pain may radiate to the shoulder, although usually not much below the upper arm. It may also radiate up into the head, usually at the back; however, in some patients it affects the forehead and eyes more than the back of the head, and then the patient may wrongly attribute the pain to chronic sinusitis.

When such patients are examined they may have limited neck movements, especially twisting movements. There is usually tenderness of the neck and shoulder muscles, which is often mainly one-sided. The muscles may feel abnormally hard.

These symptoms are almost the same and those described as typical of cervical spondylosis. This similarity is not accidental: the two disorders do give rise to very similar symptoms, and indeed the same patient may well suffer from both at the same time. Often, though not always, patients will recognize that there is a clear association between their neck symptoms and psychological tension.

It is not certain why some patients suffer in this way. One theory is that the tensing of the neck muscles is a reflex action in response to a threat, which has been programmed into our nervous system during evolution; it has the effect of protecting the vulnerable neck against an anticipated blow. If this is the case, people may tense their muscles in this way in response to real or imagined threats, even though these are not of a physical nature.

Patients with this complaint who have spondylotic changes on x-ray are often told that these explain their symptoms. But do they? The x-ray findings may be partly or wholly irrelevant – for people over the age of forty are very likely to have x-ray changes of cervical spondylosis in any case. It is therefore difficult to give a simple answer to the question of what is causing the pain in an individual person.

It can also be difficult to treat patients who suffer in this way. Pain-relieving drugs seldom help much. Physical methods of treatment, such as manipulation or acupuncture, may give the best short-term results, but the symptoms tend to recur unless the patient can come to terms with the underlying psychological tension. Some form of relaxation or meditation may be the best answer here, or regular physical exercise, which has a natural tranquillizing effect.

An interesting feature of these cases is that treating the tense muscles by physical means such as acupuncture or massage may sometimes produce striking psychological effects. The mood of the patient often improves, and occasionally they laugh or cry for several hours after the treatment has been completed without knowing why; it is as if some kind of emotional 'block' had been dissolved.

The chest region (thoracic spine)

There are several subdivisions of this region that can be sites of pain.

The thoracic outlet

The region at the base of the neck, where the neck and thorax join, is a place traversed by numerous important arteries, veins, and nerves – as well as by the windpipe and gullet. This makes it vulnerable. Moreover, the neck is a very mobile region, whereas the thorax is relatively fixed, so the place where they join is subject to a lot of mechanical stress. Pressure can arise here owing to the presence of an extra rib (cervical), or it may be due to one of the muscles (anterior scalene muscle). Pain usually begins in the shoulder, and spreads progressively down the arm to the hand, especially if the arm is used repetitively, for example in polishing. Weakness and wasting of the hands also occurs, and may replace pain as the most obvious symptoms. There may be numbness of the hands. All these symptoms are usually worse at night.

An important source of confusion here is a disorder known as the carpal tunnel syndrome. In this, a band of fibrous tissue at the front of the wrist (which serves to hold the tendons in place) compresses a major nerve to the hand, causing numbness and weakness. It is possible to relieve this pressure by dividing the band of tissue surgically, so it is essential to distinguish symptoms arising at the wrist in this way from those due at compression at the base of the neck. Usually this can be done by means of nerve conduction tests (see p. 54), although a simple clinical test that may give the answer is to press on the median nerve at the front of the wrist: if this causes the characteristic tingling in the affected fingers the diagnosis is probably carpal tunnel syndrome.

The scapula

This is a common site of pain, which may be felt along the inner border of the bone or in other areas. Sometimes the pain is referred from the spine, but in other cases it seems to be due to trigger points in the numerous muscles in this region.

The upper chest

Particularly in middle-aged women, one often sees a considerable degree of fixity in the upper part of the thoracic spine. The shoulders are rounded and the upper thoracic vertebrae and the ribs move hardly at all. These patients complain of a constant aching across the shoulders and upper back, and movements of the shoulders and arms are restricted, so that lifting things off a shelf or hanging up a dress is difficult.

The mid and lower chest

Pain originating in the spine in this region may be referred forwards in the chest, along the lines of the ribs. Pain may be felt at the tips of the ribs, or anywhere in the chest wall. Sometimes it is very severe, and it can be confused with pain due to heart disease (angina pectoris). Pain arising in the lower part of the thoracic spine, together with pain coming from the lumbar spine, can cause abdominal pain, which likewise may lead to diagnostic difficulties.

Another cause of pain in this area is shingles (herpes zoster). This gives rise to pain radiating round the back which may be very severe. Once the characteristic rash appears the diagnosis is easy, but before that it may be difficult. Shingles can affect any nerve in the body, but the commonest area is the thorax; next comes the face.

Disc prolapse occurs in the thoracic spine, as it does in the cervical and lumbar regions, and is another cause for sudden severe pain radiating round one side of the chest. It is made worse by coughing and sneezing, and sometimes even by breathing. The main anxiety about thoracic disc prolapse is that there may be pressure on the spinal cord. This can cause weakness in the legs and disturbance of bladder function: retention of urine or urgency, or a sensation of incomplete emptying. These symptoms, though fortunately rare, are an indication for urgent surgery.

The back and pelvic regions (lumbar spine and sacrum)

This region of the back gives rise to more symptoms than any other. It is also very complicated; at least 26 causes of pain here have been described. There are many possible ways in which symptoms can appear; there are variations according to age.

Lumbar back pain in young people

This seems to be increasing in frequency. Most cases occur in teenagers, especially at about the age of fourteen. The causes include prolapsed disc, vertebral fractures, spondylolisthesis, and scoliosis. Boys are affected more than girls, probably because they go in for more aggressive sports. Back problems in children cause fewer symptoms than in adults, but there are more obvious physical changes (spasm, weakness, loss of reflexes).

Patients in their early twenties

These people are often tall. The pain may be quite severe, or it may be merely a mild ache across the lower back and perhaps radiating into the buttocks or thighs. It is often worse in certain positions: sometimes sitting, sometimes standing, sometimes in bed. A common finding is that the patient (usually a young woman) stands with an exaggerated hollow in the lumbar spine (lordosis); if she places her back against the wall a considerable gap appears between the wall and her lower back. Women typically find their symptoms are worse at period times.

Movements are usually normal or nearly so, there may be little local tenderness in the back, and the legs are normal, with no radiation of pain below the knees.

Patients in this group are often said to have 'postural' pain, because poor posture seems to be an important cause of their problems.

Back pain after pelvic surgery

Women who have had gynaecological surgery, such as a hysterectomy, may begin to suffer from lumbar backache after the operation; sometimes it begins almost immediately. The cause is not always clear, but probably in many cases the patient has been placed in an abnormal posture while under the anaesthetic, with muscles relaxed, and this has caused a strain on the back structures. This kind of pain can persist for many years if untreated. Fortunately, it often responds to physical treatment such as acupuncture or osteopathy.

Spondylolisthesis

Older women, and to a lesser extent men, may suffer from chronic lumbosacral pain for months or years on end, due to spondylolisthesis. The fourth to fifth lumbar segment is the most common site for this; the fourth lumbar vertebra moves backwards and forwards more than normal.

Typically, such patients suffer from low back pain and also pain in the buttocks and thighs. It is more or less constant, but there may also be episodes when the symptoms become more severe. Both sides are often affected though one is usually worse than the other. On examining these patients, the doctor typically finds tenderness over one or two lumbar vertebrae, the sacroiliac joints, and the muscles of the lower back; there is also very often tenderness of the buttock muscles, due to the activation of trigger points. The normal curvature of the lumbar spine tends to be lost (the back is flatter than normal). However, stiffness of the back is not usually obvious, and many patients can touch their toes quite easily.

Standing for long is usually painful, but so too is sitting for long in one position.

Chronic stress backache

This tends to affect men more than women, especially strongly built stocky men with a protuberant abdomen who are used to performing heavy work. The traditional appearance of John Bull illustrates the typical patient. These patients experience pain in the middle and lower back, radiating to the flanks, buttock and groin; there is no sciatica. It begins gradually, and once established is pretty well continuous. The patient is prevented from working by his pain.

Backache and sciatica

This may begin fairly suddenly, within three or four hours of some kind of physical stress (which may be as trivial as a misstep in coming off a kerb), or it may come on more gradually. The apparent cause may be unwonted physical activity of some kind, such as the first episode of digging in the garden in spring or shovelling snow in winter, and another common story is onset after a long drive in the car. Immediately after this stress there is mild lumbar aching, but it does not seem to be too severe and a hot bath appears to relieve it.

Usually within a day or two, but sometimes later, the backache returns and is now much more severe. The lumbar muscles are in spasm and the patient may find that he cannot put on his socks or tie his shoe laces – not so much because of pain but because his lumbar spine is absolutely locked in position.

Either immediately or after a few days sciatica comes on: pain begins to be felt in one or other buttock or thigh, and may spread down the leg as far as the foot. The backache often lessens in intensity at this time and the spasm eases off sufficiently to allow the patient to touch his feet again. The leg may feel cold, and there are often strange sensations such as pins and needles or numbness. Weakness of the leg muscles may occur, and tendon reflexes may be lost. At a later stage the muscles of the affected leg may actually begin to waste away.

The doctor is likely to find that 'straight-leg raising' – the angle to which it is possible to lift the patient's affected leg from the couch – is reduced. This is because lifting the leg in this way stretches the sciatic nerve. Sometimes, however, it is the femoral nerve (at the front of the thigh) rather than the sciatic nerve that is being pressed on. In this case, the leg can be lifted upwards but not moved backwards and the patient may find it impossible to stand up straight.

On the basis of the patient's symptoms and the doctor's findings on examination a doctor may be able to state with a fair degree of confidence which level of the spine has been affected. However, this is not invariably the case, because more than one level of the spine may be involved, or the way in which the symptoms appear may not correspond to any textbook description.

It is also possible to have sciatica without backache.

Neurogenic claudication

This refers to a peculiar kind of pain which is due to narrowing of the spinal canal in the lumbar region – for example by spondylosis. The patients find that they experience unpleasant feelings in their legs, which they describe as numbness, coldness, burning or cramp. These can amount to actual pain. The characteristic feature is that the symptoms come on when the patients stand upright, especially if they walk, and are relieved by bending forwards. (For this reason some patients find they can cycle comfortably although walking is painful (see pp. 96–7). This disorder is rather similar to the much commoner one known as intermittent claudication, which is due to narrowing of the arteries in the legs. One point of difference is that patients with intermittent claudication prefer to walk downhill, because this is less demanding, while patients with neurogenic claudication prefer to walk uphill, because then they bend forwards slightly; walking downhill, in contrast, makes them lean back and so narrows their spinal canal still further.

Pregnancy

Pregnancy is not of course a disease but a normal state. Nevertheless many pregnant women do experience backache, especially towards the end of pregnancy. There are several possible reasons for this.

The most obvious is the extra stress that is imposed on the back. The weight of the baby in the uterus causes the woman to lean backwards when standing and walking, and consequently there is strain on the ligaments in the lumbar region. This effect is sometimes made worse because, as part of the preparation that the body makes for delivery, the ligaments themselves become softer and more elastic; this is an adaptation to allow the pelvis to stretch a little to make more room for the baby's head. A third factor is that the muscles of the abdominal wall stretch and may lose their tone to some extent.

Many women find that a pregnancy belt or corset relieves part of their back discomfort. But it is also important to maintain the tone and strength of the back and abdominal muscles during the early part of pregnancy, before too much enlargement has occurred; once this has happened exercise becomes difficult.

After delivery the ligaments gradually resume their normal state, but this does not happen immediately so it is important not to lift heavy weights or exert other strains on the back and pelvis at this time, otherwise the woman may be left with a degree of permanent laxity that will cause pain. Exercises after delivery will also help to restore normal tone to the muscles.

Menstruation

There is no reason why normal menstruation should cause pain in the back. Pain may be referred to the back if the periods are painful (dysmenorrhoea), and if there is any source of pain in the back it is more likely to be troublesome at this time; many women find that their pain threshold is lower.

The role of the central nervous system: the pain experience

So far, we have been looking at back pain as if it were simply to be explained in mechanical terms; by the interaction of bones, muscles, ligaments, blood vessels and nerves. And up to a point, this is reasonable; much back pain can be so explained. But, if we confine our attention to these things, we neglect some of the most important aspects of the matter.

The back, after all, is not an isolated entity, it is part of a complete organism, a human being; and that human being, in turn, is not isolated but is part of society. When we suffer back pain, we do not do so in the relatively uncomplicated manner of a dog or a horse; we bring to the situation our fears and our hopes, our previous experiences of illness and pain – right from earliest childhood, from our beliefs derived from our upbringing and from the ideas of earlier generations. All these things influence how we feel and how we behave.

One person will try to ignore the pain and disability as much as possible and will do his or her best to continue with ordinary life with the minimum interruption. Another will become chronically fearful of a recurrence of back pain, and even after recovery will attend anxiously to every little twinge, terrified in case it heralds a relapse. Superimposed on these differences in attitude are differences in people's sensitivity to pain – their so-called pain threshold. And even this pain threshold is not a fixed value, nor constant for a given person. An injury received in battle or on the playing field may cause little or no pain at the time, whereas a less serious injury in other circumstances may be excruciating.

Some people appear to respond to unhappiness and depression by experiencing pain, even in the absence of any discernible physical abnormality. The low back seems often to be a site where pain of this kind is felt. It can be difficult for patients to accept that pain is psychologically caused, but this undoubtedly is the case at times.

One reason why patients often reject explanations of this kind is that they themselves, and often their doctors, regard this 'non-organic' or 'functional' pain as somehow not quite respectable, or even as unreal. It is, however, quite as real as pain caused in other ways and may indeed be very severe.

Part of the problem comes from the fact that we often think of the mind as somehow separate from our bodies. If we picture our mind as something like the driver of a car, to suffer from 'functional' pain becomes something like being a bad driver. The car itself is working perfectly well, so if anything is wrong it must be the fault of the driver.

In order to understand how pain is felt, we would do better to forget about the driver–car analogy altogether, and instead to picture the whole organism – back structures, brain and spinal cord, *and* conscious mind – as forming one complete unit.

Modern conceptions of how pain is perceived within the central nervous system correspond with this 'holistic' way of thinking. The old idea of pain perception was that injury to an external part of the body – stepping on a drawing pin, say – would send a 'pain impulse' up the nerves to the spinal cord and thence to the brain, where it would be registered in a supposed 'pain centre'.

It now appears, however, that there is no 'pain centre' as such. There are parts of the brain that have maps to record vision, hearing, touch and so forth, but there is no corresponding area for pain. So how is pain felt?

A detailed answer to this question would take us into very deep waters indeed, and at present we are not able to explain the matter anything like fully. But perhaps we could think of it by analogy with a malfunctioning radio.

If a radio is overloaded it may begin to utter a piercing howl. It does not do this by design; the manufacturer has not placed a special 'howling component' in the mechanism, to indicate that it is not functioning properly. Rather, the howl is a consequence of over-amplification of electrical activity by a form of 'positive feedback'.

Pain could perhaps be thought of as a kind of 'howl' within the central nervous system. It can occur when the system is overloaded in various ways.

We are often told that pain is a useful warning, and of course this is often true. It makes us avoid damaging influences such as excessive heat and cold, and it prevents us from using injured limbs until they have healed. But much pain is useless, and it may also be excessive for the 'intended' effect. Does toothache, for example, need to be *quite* so severe? And what about the pain that persists long after the original injury has healed, or that which occurs without any apparent injury at all?

An important notion that helps to explain some of these things is the idea of 'pain memory'. The word 'memory' is used in a special sense here. It does not refer to the thought of pain, which may come into one's mind as one recalls lying in bed with an acute attack of sciatica. Instead, it denotes the persistence of a trace of some kind within the central nervous system (probably in many cases in the spinal cord).

When the body is injured in any way there is usually a certain amount of pain, which is felt at the site of injury and is roughly proportionate to the severity of the injury. As the injury heals the pain normally gets better and disappears.

Sometimes, however, for reasons that are not clear, the pain does not disappear when the injury heals but instead persists for weeks, months, or even years. When confronted with a patient in whom this has happened doctors generally look for some kind of persisting change at the site of injury, but this can seldom be found. It seems, therefore, that what happens in such cases is a long-lasting change within the central nervous system itself. We do not know what this change is; it could be the establishment of a self-perpetuating circuit of nerve impulses, or perhaps a chemical alteration in some cells. Acupuncture may act by 'turning off' central nervous systems of this kind.

It is possible that many cases of persistent back pain are due to this 'pain memory', especially those in which investigations fail to show any convincing cause in the back itself. It follows that operations and other measures directed at the spine will fail in such cases, but acupuncture, manipulation, and transcutaneous electrical nerve stimulation (TENS), all of which appear to alter the patterns of nerve impulses entering the central nervous system, sometimes succeed.

The underlying idea is that, once a particular pattern of excitation has occurred within the central nervous systen, it tends to perpetuate itself, and either to go on all the time or to be called back into activity by a stimulus of any kind. It is like a well-worn path; later arrivals follow it automatically. An injury of any kind, including damage to some of the back structures, can set up a pattern of activity in the central nervous system that gives rise to the subjective experience of pain. Even after the original injury has been repaired, the central nervous system can continue to reproduce this pattern and so pain can still be felt.

Of course, this does not always happen; but we naturally ask why it does happen sometimes. And yet perhaps this is the wrong question; perhaps we ought to ask why it doesn't always happen. In other words, what normally turns these pain patterns off once the injury has healed?

Although the answer to this question is not fully known, part of the explanation seems to be that pain patterns are turned off by activity in other parts of the nervous system. This activity sends impulses into the central nervous system that have the effect of blocking or deactivating the pain patterns. Probably this is in part explains how treatments such as acupuncture, osteopathy and exercise can help to relieve pain. Some neurologists believe that the reason why pressure on a nerve root causes pain may not be that this sends abnormal impulses into the central nervous system, but rather that it *blocks* the beneficial impulses needed to prevent pain.

In summary, then, there are two possible ways of accounting for pain as a phenomenon. One idea is that it is a kind of subjective side-effect produced by the mechanisms that are responsible for inflammation or repair. The other is that pain is always waiting in the wings, so to speak, but that, under normal circumstances it is continuously suppressed. There is possibly some truth in both these ideas. In any case, the important thing to understand is that because pain is 'produced' by the central nervous system, which is also responsible for maintaining consciousness, psychological attitudes are always important in pain. How we think about our experience of pain can alter that experience quite profoundly, and it is even possible to have pain that is produced entirely psychologically.

The role of conscious attitude in pain perception

If we avoid thinking of the mind as a driver in a car, and think of it instead as a function of the activity within the brain, we can begin to understand how it can affect the way in which pain is felt in back disease. It is known that the 'higher centres' in the brain can modify the activity of the spinal cord. This isn't a matter of 'imagination', or 'mind over matter', but rather of how the nervous system as a whole operates.

If we think of things in this way it becomes easier to understand how, say, depression, can cause back pain. There are undoubtedly chemical and electrical changes in the brain in some cases of depression. This doesn't necessarily mean that depression is wholly a physical illness, like pneumonia, but it points to the fact that physical and psychological factors are so mixed up with each other that it is often impossible to disentangle them. And because these physical changes occur in the brain, it is hardly surprising that there should also be physical changes in the spinal cord, too, which is, after all, an extension of the brain.

It is therefore easy to understand in principle, if not in detail, why depression can cause backache. Investigations of the back in depressed people do not show anything wrong; this is hardly surprising, because there is nothing wrong at that level. There is little point in going on and on looking for a physical explanation for the pain, because follow-up studies have repeatedly shown that if nothing abnormal is found initially it is extremely unlikely that a serious physical problem will be discovered later. Physical changes of a kind have occurred, but they are at the level of the brain and spinal cord, and these are not detectable by present methods of examination. But the important thing to understand is that the pain is perfectly real – just as real, in fact, as the pain of a prolapse disc or fractured vertebra.

It follows from this, of course, that treatment directed at the back itself will be useless in such cases. What is needed is treatment of the depression, which may be by antidepressant drugs, by psycho-therapy, or by some kind of change in the patient's attitude and expectations – cognitive therapy (see pp. 82–3).

By no means all patients whose symptoms are primarily psychological have an identifiable psychological disorder, such as depression. In most cases a whole range of mental and emotional factors is involved, and of course there is nothing to say that a patient whose problems are mainly psychological may not also have some minor physical problems in the back as well. In general, there is seldom just one explanation for these patients' symptoms.

The converse of all this is also true. Even when there is a clearly identifiable physical cause for a patient's back pain, there will almost inevitably be psychological effects which will tend to hasten or retard recovery. Again, this happens not by superimposing an 'imaginary' layer on the underlying physical illness, but by modify-ing the way in which the central nervous system behaves. If someone suffering from acute backache is excessively anxious about what is happening at work in his absence, or is terrified that he will be incapacitated for months or years, these fears will tend to make his pain worse by a direct effect on the central nervous system.

For those unfortunate persons whose pain fails to respond to any kind of treatment, the best plan is to investigate strategies for coping with the pain as it is; some pain clinics in this country are exploring ways of doing this (see p. 82).

4

Coping With Back Pain I:
Treatments

How you react to your back pain will depend, among other things, on whether this is your first attack or a recurrence. If you are familiar with your pain you will have some idea of how it is likely to develop, but if it is your first experience you may well feel considerable alarm.

A first attack

What to do

The first thing is not to panic. Remember that the vast majority of people (about 90 per cent) recover from their back pain within a few weeks, and some recover much sooner.

If the pain is severe, you should go to bed and lie down. Sometimes this may be difficult: if you are completely unable to straighten up, as may happen, all you can do is to lower yourself cautiously to the floor without altering the angle of your back. In any case you should avoid repeating the movement that brought on your pain – if you know what it was.

Having got to bed, you should adopt whatever position you find most comfortable. There is no rule about this, although lying flat on your back or flat on your front are unlikely to be good ideas because these positions place a strain on the back. Lying on one side is often best, with a pillow between your knees to prevent your upper thigh from pulling you over and twisting your spine. Whatever position you adopt, the ideal is to keep your whole spine as level as possible; cushions and pillows should be used to achieve this effect.

Turning over in bed may be difficult. It is often easiest to draw your knees up, and then to allow the weight of your legs to pull you over, without twisting your spine. It helps to do this if you avoid having heavy bedclothes on your legs; it is better to keep the room warm and use only a light cover if possible. Try to work out a routine of turning which minimizes the twisting action of your spine.

Helpful friends or relatives are likely to suggest that your bed is not hard enough, and may want to place boards underneath your mattress to make it rigid. As a rule this is not necessary; a very hard bed may indeed be more uncomfortable than a softer one. Provided your bed does not actually sag it should be satisfactory as it is.

Occasionally someone finds that lying down, in any position, is actually more painful than sitting. In this case it is obviously better to sit.

Getting to the lavatory may be a problem. Provided a lavatory is within reasonable distance of your bed and on the same floor, it is best to try to use it rather than attempt alternative arrangements. Bed pans and so forth, even if they are available, have more disadvantages than benefits for most people.

It is likely that you will be constipated for the first few days, partly because of the pain, partly from lack of exercise, and possibly as a result of some of the medicines you may be given for pain. There is no need to do anything; it will sort itself out later.

Pain relief

You should take some form of pain-relieving tablet. Aspirin or paracetamol, or any other proprietory product that you favour, is likely to be helpful; it should be taken in the maximum permissible dosage, although this should not be exceeded. Some people find a source of local warmth such as a hot water bottle helpful. Perhaps rather surprisingly, cold applications can also give relief; a bag of frozen peas is often suggested. However, it is possible to suffer skin burns from cold as well as from heat; to prevent this, apply some Vaseline or a damp towel to the skin before applying the ice-pack and do not leave it in position for more than about 15 or 20 minutes at a time. Massage by a friend or relative may also be soothing, but it should be gentle, with some lubricating cream (e.g. baby oil or lotion) being used to prevent chafing of the skin. There is no need to use any proprietory 'pain-relieving' cream although it will not cause any harm if you do.

Pain relieving creams are of two kinds. Some, which can be bought over the counter, contain minor skin irritants that produce a feeling of local warmth due to an increase in blood flow. This may give some pain relief by a counter-irritant effect. Probably what happens is that an increase in the number of nerve impulses coming from the skin reduces the ability of the central nervous system to register the pain from the deep structures in the back.

A second type of cream contains anti-inflammatory drugs similar to aspirin. Creams of this kind are available only on prescription. It is unlikely that they can have any direct local effect on the spine, since this is too deep for the drug to reach from the skin, the drug is absorbed into the blood stream from the skin, but the effect is little different from what it would be if the same substance had been taken by mouth.

If you can obtain a TENS machine (see p. 56) this may afford good relief.

Calling your doctor

Provided there is no loss of bladder function (a very rare complication) or severe sciatica there is no need to call your doctor in immediately. Wait for three days and see how you get on. If you are beginning to recover by then you can make an appointment at the surgery, since you will probably need a sickness certificate for your work. If there is no sign of recovery in three days, or if you have developed significant sciatica, it is advisable to see your doctor.

All these remarks refer to fairly severe backache, which leaves you with little choice but to go to bed. The position as regards less severe, relatively minor back pain is less clear-cut. It is not certain that going to bed and resting really shortens the duration of the pain, and it may be preferable to keep going, perhaps with the help of pain-relieving tablets, if that is reasonably possible. Once again, however, you should see your doctor, especially in a first attack, if there has been no improvement within a few days.

When you see your doctor

If you do see your doctor, he or she will ask you about your symptoms and whether you have had similar attacks before. Next will probably come an examination: you will be asked to undress, and then the doctor will look at your back, test your range of movements, and press your back in various places to see if it is tender. The doctor will probably also examine your abdomen in case there is anything that could be referring pain to your spine; if you are a middle-aged or elderly man your prostate gland may be examined as well (via the rectum) as cancer of the prostate can cause back pain. The strength of your legs will probably be tested, together with your tendon reflexes, which are often impaired or lost in sciatica. Raising each leg off the couch in turn helps to show whether there is pressure on the sciatic nerve; although this test usually forms part of the examination, the information it provides is not always very helpful.

On the basis of all this your doctor may be able to make a diagnosis, or at least an educated guess about the likely cause of your problem. However, he may want to arrange for some investigations; the likely ones are a blood test and an x-ray of the spine.

X-rays

It is important for you to understand what these tests can and cannot show. The main reason for doing them is to exclude the uncommon but serious causes of back pain, such as cancer. Certain other diseases, such as ankylosing spondylitis or severe osteoporosis, will probably also show up if they are present, and so will spondylolisthesis. However, prolapsed discs or 'trapped nerves' are not shown adequately by a plain x-ray. True, an x-ray may show 'disc space narrowing', which indicates that some disc material has escaped at some time in the past, and it may show other features such as osteoarthrosis, but it cannot prove that these features, even if they are present, are the cause of your symptoms. More specialized investigations (discussed below) are needed for this.

What follows from this is that repeated x-rays for recurrent episodes of back pain are seldom necessary or desirable. They do not help in treatment, and modern practice is to cut down the number of x-rays as much as possible so as to limit their possible adverse effects.

If the medications you have used so far have not provided adequate pain relief your doctor may prescribe something stronger. It is at this stage that the question of seeing a specialist usually comes up.

When to see a specialist

The vast majority of patients recover from back pain with simple first-aid treatment of the kind just outlined; it is not usually necessary to do anything further. However, if there is no significant improvement in your symptoms after a few weeks, or if residual pain or weakness persists after about three months, your doctor may decide that you ought to see a specialist, who may be either a neurologist or an orthopaedic surgeon. Referral to a pain clinic is also possible, but probably not at this stage. Pain clinics are run by anaesthetists, and patients are usually referred to them only when all the ordinary back investigations and treatments have been tried and found to have failed.

Seeing a specialist

To start with the specialist will repeat the same kind of procedure that your own doctor has already carried out: he or she will take a history and examine you. The clinical examination may be more detailed on this occasion. The specialist will probably check your posture standing as well as lying down, and he or she may also look at how you walk and how you get undressed, because all this can give an indication of the amount of disability you are suffering from. Any difficulty you experience in turning over on the examination couch may also be important.

Further blood tests may be carried out and, if an x-ray has not yet been done by your own doctor, it probably will be ordered now. In addition, the specialist will have at his disposal some more elaborate forms of investigation, some or all of which he may order for you.

In describing your symptoms to the specialist, try to confine yourself to what you actually feel and avoid offering a diagnosis. It is not helpful for you to use terms like 'inflammation' or 'congestion' since the reason you have come to the specialist is to decide what the diagnosis is. Be aware, also, that what you understand by descriptive terms may be different from what the doctor understands. To the doctor, for example, 'numbness' implies a partial or complete loss of sensation, but some patients use it to indicate weakness or other inability to use a limb. It is important to make sure that you and the doctor both know what you are talking about.

Quality of pain is often hard to describe; words such as throbbing, burning, sharp and dull seem to mean different things to different people and so are not always very helpful. But notice particularly which parts of your back or leg are most affected, the changes in position or activity (standing, sitting, lying down; walking, driving; coughing and sneezing) that make the pain better or worse, together with any associated symptoms such as pins and needles or impairment of sensation. Times at which the pain is worse can sometimes be helpful. Also be prepared to give a clear account of how and when the symptoms first appeared and the changes that have occurred in them subsequently; and make a mental note of the relief, or absence of relief, that you have experienced from taking any medicines or other treatment that has been prescribed.

Special investigations

Myelography or radiculography

As mentioned already, a plain x-ray can show the bones and the gaps between them (the joint spaces), but it does not show the actual discs or nerve roots. For many years the standard way of doing this was to inject a liquid into the spinal canal at a level below the first lumbar vertebra, where the spinal cord ends. The liquid is opaque to x-rays and so if something is pressing on a nerve root it will show up as an indentation. Some of the fluid that bathes the spinal cord and brain (cerebrospinal fluid) is drawn off for examination at the same time. This procedure is called myelography.

The radiologist will inject the radioopaque dye and then you will be tilted in various directions so that the way the dye flows in the spine can be seen on a screen. Films of the appearance of the spine are also taken from different angles.

As a variant on myelography, the liquid may be injected selectively into the dura mater sheaths surrounding the nerve roots (radiculography).

Although myelography is still used, it is often replaced today by one of the newer investigations discussed below. Patients generally find myelography fairly unpleasant, and although the risk of inflammation of the arachnoid lining has now been reduced by changing the liquid used from an oil-based to a water-based one, patients may still experience headache or nausea immediately after the examination and they need to be kept lying down, usually overnight, to reduce this as much as possible.

Discography

This is a form of examination in which x-ray-opaque liquid is injected directly into an intervertebral disc in order to show whether it is pressing on surrounding structures. The technique is not very widely used.

Scans

Computerized axial tomography (CAT or CT) scans and magnetic resonance imaging (MRI) are relatively new techniques that can produce astonishingly detailed pictures of the structures of the spine, including the discs and nerves. Moreover, they are pain-free and almost entirely safe, CAT (or CT) scanning does use x-rays but the dosage is small; MRI scanning does not use x-rays and is entirely safe so far as is known.

Computerized axial tomography is a method of enhancing the appearance and accuracy of x-rays by combining a series of views from different angles with the help of a computer. It takes about twenty minutes to perform but is not unpleasant, though it may also be combined with myelography.

Magnetic resonance imaging does not use x-rays; instead, the patient is placed in a very strong magnetic field, which however cannot be felt. This causes the nuclei of the atoms in the body to orientate themselves in a particular direction; when the magnetic field is switched off they lose this orientation and the rate at which they do so is measured. Different tissues change at varying rates and this difference is used to build up a picture of the structures in the body.

MRI scanning is still at a fairly early stage in its development and the apparatus is extremely expensive, so it is not widely available.

Ultrasound

This is a technique in which high-frequency sound is used to generate a picture; different tissues reflect the sound in varying ways. Ultrasound is, again, safe so far as is known, but although it is widely used for examining the heart and the pelvic organs in women its role in back pain is fairly limited at present. It can, however, be used to measure the diameter of the spinal canal in the lumbar region, to see whether there is significant narrowing that may press on the nerve roots in that area (see p. 22).

Electromyography

Electromyography (EMG) is a technique for recording the electrical activity of the muscles. It is sometimes used to investigate the efficiency with which the nerves are conducting impulses; fine needles are inserted into the muscles, but it is not especially painful.

Treatments

Depending on the results of his or her examination and of the investigations ordered, the specialist will decide what treatment to offer you. There are a number of possibilities; it is important that you understand what treatment may be intended to achieve.

Purposes of treatment

Relief of pain

This is normally the primary purpose of treatment, since pain is naturally the main preoccupation of the sufferer. Until pain has been relieved – or at least contained – there is little point in going further.

Restoration of normal movement

This includes freeing joints and other structures the range of movement of which may have become restricted (passive movement), and of improving the strength of muscles that have become weak (active movement).

Stabilization

This is the elimination of weakness and abnormal movements that may predispose to subsequent relapses.

Postural correction

The restoration of the normal position of bones is desirable as far as possible.

Restoration of function

Improvement of confidence, elimination of faulty habits at home and at work, advice about care of the back, are all important treatment objectives.

Not all these objectives are applicable in every case, and even when they are, the extent to which they can be achieved varies considerably from patient to patient.

Drugs

The medicines used for back pain include all those also used for the treatment of rheumatic disorders. The prototype of this group is aspirin, but there is a range of newer drugs which have broadly similar effects to aspirin; they are called non-steroidal anti-inflammatory drugs (NSAIDs). They are effective for many people though they may have side-effects, notably on the stomach, where they can cause ulceration, particularly if taken without food or milk. For this reason some patients are unable to take them at all; if you are intolerant of one drug in this group you should not take any of the others. If a patient is intolerant of NSAIDs it may sometimes be possible to counteract this by giving another drug at the same time to protect the stomach; otherwise it will be necessary to substitute a drug from a different group, but there are not too many of these.

Patients vary considerably in their response to the different drugs; some people may get no help from one kind but do very well with another. Although they are called anti-inflammatory drugs, their main use in back pain is as pain relievers. They do not cure the disorder but keep the symptoms at bay until natural recovery occurs.

Transcutaneous electrical nerve stimulation

Transcutaneous electrical nerve stimulation (TENS) is often used today in pain clinics. It has a good deal in common with acupuncture, and may indeed work in much the same way (see pp. 68–73). Many pain clinics now offer acupuncture as well. The treatment may be given either by a doctor or by a physiotherapist.

The idea of using electricity to relieve pain is an old one; the Romans, it appears, advocated standing on an electric eel for the purpose. The modern apparatus consists of a small battery-operated machine, about the size of a cigarette packet, from which run two or four wires connected to conducting rubber pads. The pads are placed on either side of the painful area or over a major nerve leading to it. In back pain, for example, they might be placed on either side of the neck, on either side of the lumbar spine, or (for sciatica) over the sciatic nerve.

Controls on the machine allow the patient to adjust the intensity of the current and also its frequency (the number of pulses it gives out per second). A fast rate (about 80 pulses per second) is usually best. The patient feels a tingling sensation under the pads; this is not normally unpleasant.

Not all patients respond to this form of treatment (somewhere between one- and two-thirds of those who try it). Of those who do respond, however, some obtain very good relief and others are helped considerably. If there is an effect, it usually appears within a few minutes of turning the machine on, and it lasts as long as the current is applied. Sometimes there is a pain-free period after the machine is turned off, but this is unusual. It follows that patients may need to wear the machine for long periods – perhaps all day or even continuously; however, they can walk about and carry on their normal activities, apart from bathing, while doing so.

TENS is very safe. Some patients suffer from skin irritation under the pads, but this can often be avoided by changing the position of the pads slightly.

TENS machines are available for loan or can be purchased outright.

Physiotherapy

Most hospitals have a physiotherapy department, staffed by state registered physiotherapists; that is, people who have studied for three or four years and have passed the examinations required for membership of the Chartered Society of Physiotherapy (MCSP). Some physiotherapists practise privately, outside the National Health Service. As the law stands at present, anyone in Britain can set himself up as a physiotherapist, but only those who have passed the examination can use the letters MCSP. It is not necessary to be referred to a private physiotherapist by a doctor, although for ethical reasons physiotherapists usually do require a letter of referral from a patient's family doctor, to whom they write a letter indicating their opinion and the treatment they recommend.

Physiotherapists use a wide range of treatment methods. A principal one is manipulation, a term which refers to a number of manual techniques ranging from gentle massage to vigorous mobilization. The massage is intended to produce relaxation and improve circulation. Mobilization techniques are intended to relieve pain and to increase the range of movement. There is a good deal of common ground between these forms of treatment and those used by osteopaths and chiropractors (see pp. 65–8). The techniques employed include regional mobilization (gentle repeated movements of the affected part of the back) and localized mobilization, directed to the spinal segment or segments that are not moving freely.

One method of manipulation that has been in use by physio-therapists for many years is traction. The idea is to stretch the spine by applying a load to it, the original assumption being that the disc would be 'drawn back' into its correct place and the alignment of the vertebrae improved. It seems unlikely that this is how traction really works; it is not possible to draw back extruded disc material in this way. Possibly the beneficial effects are due to changes in the muscles or to reduction of partial dislocation (subluxation) of facet joints.

Traction can be applied in many different ways, but generally a harness of some kind is attached to the patient and traction is applied for up to 20 minutes or so; occasionally patients are admitted to hospital for more prolonged traction. The pull used is heavier for the lumbar spine than for the neck. Relief of pain during traction may occur but is not of much significance. However, a significant number of patients get long-lasting relief from the treatment and this is worth while.

Some patients use apparatus at home to give themselves traction. A simple method is to hang by the arms from a door or similar support, although the patient must have fairly strong hands to do this and a strong door is also required. More elaborate apparatus consists of frames which hold the patient and tilt to produce traction by gravity. Such methods should only be used on medical advice, since for some people it is unsafe to increase the blood pressure in the head and eyes by adopting a head-down posture.

Exercises may be used, either individually or in groups (the 'back school' approach). In a typical back school, six patients are given instruction over four sessions by a physiotherapist. The idea is to increase the patients' understanding of their problem, to allow them to meet fellow-sufferers, to teach them how to use their backs with greater efficiency and less strain, and to strengthen the abdominal muscles as a protection against further damage to the back. As well as the psychological support that meeting in a group provides for patients, this method obviously helps in coping with the huge numbers of patients who suffer from back symptoms.

Whether patients are seen singly or in groups, they may be shown exercises to do at home (see p. 94 and following for a selection of these).

Physiotherapists may employ a variety of electrical and physical methods of stimulation. Ultrasound – high frequency sound – applies energy to the deep tissues (muscles, tendons, ligaments) and helps to reduce pain and swelling, mainly in the treatment of acute pain. Short-wave and microwave therapy use electromagnetic energy to produce similar effects. Interferential therapy, which has something in common with TENS, applies electrical energy to the tissues through the skin.

Collars, corsets, and other appliances

The consultant or a physiotherapist may also suggest other measures, such as the use of a collar (for neck pain) or a corset. These do not cure the disorder but some patients find them helpful, perhaps because they limit the amount of movement in the neck or back.

Collars are generally made of latex sponge rubber or similar material. Hard collars made of plastic are also used at times but are less comfortable. Whatever the material, the collar should be individually fitted to the patient. The main reasons for using a collar are to support the head and prevent movements which make the pain worse, to prevent jarring of the neck while driving, and to relieve pain that comes on while the patient is asleep.

Lumbar supports come in a bewildering variety of shapes and sizes. At one extreme there is the plaster-of-paris jacket, and at the other a simple affair consisting of little more than an elasticated belt; in between are various designs of corsets reinforced with steel or plastic struts.

It is difficult to be sure what corsets do – or fail to do. For some people they have a strong placebo effect – they make them feel better for psychological reasons – although others instinctively reject the idea of wearing a corset. Probably the main benefit of a corset is that it raises the pressure inside the abdomen. Research has shown, perhaps rather surprisingly, that this can decrease the load on the intervertebral discs and reduce the pressure in these by as much as 30 per cent.

Another way of increasing pressure inside the abdomen is to improve the strength and tone of the abdominal muscles (see p. 103). Patients are often advised not to wear a corset for too long in case it makes their abdominal muscles weak. However, there is no real evidence that this happens; research suggests that there is no weakening even after a corset has been worn for several years. Nevertheless it is better not to become dependent on any kind of apparatus if it can be avoided.

The surgeon may prescribe a corset to be worn for a time after an operation.

If your backache is thought to be due to a short leg on one side you may be advised to wear a heel lift on the short side. Some patients develop one-sided pain when sitting, owing to inequality between the two sides of the pelvis; in such cases a small cushion placed under one buttock may help.

Minor surgical procedures

Epidural injection

This is a form of treatment in which local anaesthetic is injected into the epidural space, between the dural tube and the spinal canal. A mixture of a corticosteroid drug and a local anaesthetic is injected either in the lumbar region or through the lower part of the sacrum, with the aim of reducing inflammation and relieving pain. It does not provide a cure, but can give relief while waiting for a natural improvement to occur. It is usually done as an outpatient procedure and patients can generally go home after 20 or 30 minutes. The pain may become worse for a day or two, and then it improves. Some patients require a second injection after one or two weeks.

Facet joint injection

Hydrocortisone is injected into the joint cavity of one or more facet joints. This procedure can give long-lasting relief.

Sclerosing injections

If the problem is thought to be instability of the joints in the back, an irritant solution may be injected into the ligaments with the aim of reducing the abnormal mobility. Some patients find this painful, but it can give relief. How it actually works is uncertain; possibly it is really another form of acupuncture (see pp. 68–74).

Nerve block

Local anaesthetic is injected to block the transmission of pain impulses in the nerves going to the painful area. One might expect that this would afford only temporary relief, but in fact the relief can be quite long-lasting.

Rhizotomy and rhizolysis

These are methods of cutting or destroying nerve roots in order to relieve pain. Patients are admitted to hospital for this, usually for 48 hours. After surgery mobilization exercises are given by a physiotherapist.

Discolysis (chemonucleolysis)

An enzyme (chymopapain) is injected into the disc, with the aim of softening the disc material and allowing it to dissolve. It is usually done under general anaesthesia. Chymopapain is derived from the paw-paw fruit and is used as a meat tenderizer; the idea of the treatment is to break down the disc material and to soften it. This technique is much less traumatic than an open operation and, if successful, the patient can resume normal life quite quickly. It is done with local anaesthesia and sometimes sedation, but not a general anaesthetic. It has been used quite a lot in the United States, but relatively few surgeons in Britain have taken it up. It is not applicable in all cases.

Major surgery

Few patients (only about 1 in 10,000) with back pain ever come to operation. Unless there is an emergency, such as instability of the atlantoaxial joint in the neck or interference with bladder function, surgery will generally only be considered if other forms of treatment have failed – and even then only if there is fairly definite evidence that something (usually, though not always, a prolapsed inter-vertebral disc) is pressing on nerve roots or (much more serious) the spinal cord. The aim of the operation will then be to remove whatever is causing the pressure. Surgery may also be used to cure instability of the spine.

Surgery may be advised for problems at any level of the spine, but operations on the lumbar spine are undertaken more commonly than on the cervical or thoracic spine because of the danger of injuring the spinal cord at these higher levels. The main reasons for undertaking surgery are to relieve compression of nerve roots and to stabilize the spine. The techniques used include laminectomy (cutting away all or part of a lamina or neural arch) and fenestration (opening the spinal canal through a window, but without cutting away bone). Disc material that has leaked out from an annulus fibrosus may be removed at operation; bone that is pressing on nerves may be cut away; and metal rods, screws or bone chips may be placed to improve the stability of the spine.

The surgeon's problem is to open the spine sufficiently to see what is going on inside, but without leaving the spine in too unstable a state afterwards. Some surgeons have therefore tried a 'micro-surgical' technique, in which only a small opening is made and the whole operation takes well under an hour.

The results of surgery can be very good – especially as regards pain, which is the main indication for doing it; there is less improvement in muscle weakness. As with any operation, there is, unfortunately, a failure rate, and some patients are not improved after operation. This poses a difficult problem for both surgeon and patient: second and even third operations are sometimes carried out but the results of re-operation are considerably worse and the technical difficulties are greater.

5

Coping with Back Pain II:
The Alternative Version

Sooner or later anyone who suffers from chronic or recurrent back pain is almost certain to be advised by friends or relatives to try some form of alternative medicine. Back pain is, indeed, one of the main disorders treated by alternative practitioners, which is perhaps hardly surprising in view of the very large number of people who suffer from this complaint, and the failure of orthodox treatments to provide relief for a considerable proportion of them. Some people may indeed think of alternative treatment as the first thing to try in an acute attack, but in these cases it is important to get an accurate diagnosis first.

Until quite recently most doctors were dismissive of unorthodox methods. But traditional and folk remedies for back pain have always existed. All of these, presumably, continue to be used because they appear to work at least some of the time. To a considerable extent this reflects the fact that most back problems clear up spontaneously, with or without treatment; in such cases, whatever treatment happens to be in use at the time tends to get the credit. If we are honest, we have to admit that much the same is true of our modern treatments. However, the introduction of the scientific method has meant that attempts are made today to verify the efficacy of treatments by means of 'controlled trials', in which the treatment in question is compared with others and the results are evaluated as objectively as possible.

These methods have been applied to some extent to some of the unconventional treatments such as osteopathy, chiropractic and acupuncture, and in general the results have been encouraging. These methods appear to work at least as well as conventional ones and in some cases better. Recently, a well-known rheumatology consultant from one of the country's leading hospitals went so far as to say that in his opinion acupuncture was the only treatment that appeared to work for sciatica. No doubt this is a slight overstatement of the position, but it does give an idea of how far the older attitude of complete rejection of anything unorthodox has changed in recent years.

The criticism that is often raised against the various kinds of unorthodox treatment is that no one knows how they work. There is some justification for this objection, but the same could be said about many of the treatments that are accepted by conventional medicine. There is no agreement, for example, about how traction works. Therefore, this does not mean that there is no need to try to study the mechanism of acupuncture, manipulation and so on, but in the meantime it is acceptable to use them on the basis that they appear to work in practice.

The distinction between conventional and alternative, or complementary, treatment for back pain is not hard and fast. Some of the techniques used by osteopaths have been adopted by physiotherapists, for example, and the use of injection therapy to relieve pain has a fair amount in common with acupuncture. Some forms of alternative medicine (acupuncture, osteopathy, homoeopathy) are used by a number of conventional doctors, and, conversely, it seems likely that osteopathy and possibly other alternative treatments will achieve state recognition in Britain in the not-too-distant future. Lectures on alternative medicine are beginning to creep into the already overcrowded curriculum at some British medical schools.

Practitioners of almost all the very numerous kinds of alternative medicine would probably claim to be able to help back pain, but in practice most patients are likely to consider trying an 'alternative' therapy from a fairly limited range. The main ones are:

- Physical methods: massage, osteopathy and chiropractice, acupuncture.
- Medical methods: homoeopathy, herbalism, naturopathy.
- Psychological or psychophysical: the Alexander technique, relaxation, meditation.

To some extent, choosing among these approaches is a matter of personal preference; obviously you are not going to consider having acupuncture if you are afraid of needles. If you have been in the habit of taking homoeopathic medicine throughout your life, as some people have, it is natural that you will turn to homoeopathy again. In general terms, however, most patients suffering from back pain will tend to think first of the 'physical' forms of treatment, and this is usually a sensible choice.

Given that you are thinking of trying alternative medicine, how should you proceed? Perhaps you already know and trust a practitioner of one of these methods. If not, however, how should you go about finding one? And should you first seek the advice of your family doctor?

Choosing a practitioner

In most cases the first step should be to ask the advice of your family doctor. Perhaps he or she, or another partner in the practice, will be using one of the alternative techniques; these days an increasing number of general practitioners have trained in homoeopathy, osteopathy, or acupuncture. If not, he or she may be able to recommend you to someone else in the neighbourhood whom they trust; this person may be medically qualified, but not necessarily so; it is no longer considered unethical for a doctor to recommend a patient to a non-medical practitioner provided the doctor retains over-all responsibility for the patient's care.

It is possible that your doctor may tell you that you are unsuitable for a particular kind of alternative treatment. There may be a good reason for this; for example, an unstable spine might be made worse by manipulation. If this is the case you should respect this advice.

It is also possible that your doctor may have a prejudice against all forms of unconventional treatment and object to your receiving any of them. If this is the case, you are entitled to make your own mind up about what course of action to pursue, but if you are strongly motivated towards alternative medicine in general it might be advisable to consider looking for a new doctor who would be more sympathetic to your ideas.

In some cases it may not be strictly necessary to ask your doctor's opinion about seeking alternative treatment. For example, if you have a long history of back pain which has been fully investigated in the past and for which you have already tried orthodox treatment without success, no harm will be done if you try an alternative approach on your own initiative. Even in this case, however, it would be better to inform your doctor of your decision, and the practitioner you consult may want to write to your family doctor to say what he or she plans to do; if this practitioner is himself a doctor, he ought to do this, although it has to be with your permission.

If you do decide to seek alternative treatment on your own initiative you may find yourself somewhat at sea owing to the bewildering variety of choice that is available, and the chance does unfortunately exist that you will be not helped or even that you will be made worse. This is because in Britain there are few legal restrictions on unconventional practitioners. As the law stands at present, anyone can advertise himself or herself as an acupuncturist, homoeopath, osteopath, or anything else, even without any kind of training at all. Untrained, unqualified practitioners of this kind obviously do not belong to any professional body which could strike them off its register in the event of malpractice, and if anything goes wrong they are not insured against claims. Patients who feel they have been wrongly treated by such a person have to seek redress under the common law – an uncertain prospect at best.

The better-established alternative therapies are making progress towards setting up governing bodies and a registration system for practitioners. Currently, the osteopaths have made the most progress along this road, but there is still some way to go. The letters MRO after someone's name indicate membership of the General Council and Register of Osteopaths, but DO (diploma in osteopathy) may refer only to a 'qualification' obtained through a correspondence course. The position as regards other forms of alternative treatment is more uncertain still.

Whenever you can, you should choose an alternative practitioner on the basis of personal recommendation from someone whose opinion you trust. Only if all else fails should you resort to picking a name at random out of the telephone directory or a similar list; if you have to do this, at least make sure that the person you choose has a recognized qualification of *some* kind.

Individual therapies

Osteopathy and chiropractic

It is convenient to group these two forms of treatment together, since although their origins are somewhat different the methods they use have a lot in common. Both originated in America: osteopathy derives from the work of a doctor, Andrew Taylor Still (1828–1912); chiropractic from that of a non-doctor, David Henry Palmer (1845–1913). The theories originally advanced to explain how the treatments work were somewhat different, and so were the manipulative techniques; chiropractors at one time used x-rays more frequently than osteopaths. The similarities, however, are more important than the differences.

As we have seen, it is possible to practise these treatments with or without formal training. Four-year courses leading to a diploma are provided for people without medical qualifications by the British School of Osteopathy, the European School of Osteopathy, and the British School of Naturopathy and Osteopathy. People who have qualified in one of these ways (or as an American doctor of osteopathy) are entitled to membership of the Register of Osteopaths (MRO). They may also be members of the British Association of Manipulative Medicine. Doctors who wish to learn osteopathy may take a one-year course at The London College of Osteopathic Medicine; this entitles them to use the letters MLCOM.

Chiropractors also study for four years in Britain or the USA, and this entitles them to membership of the British Chiropractors' Association.

Naturopaths also use manipulation as part of a wider approach involving diet and various changes in lifestyle. Practitioners who have trained for four years at the British College of Naturopathy and Osteopathy use the letters ND or DO and may become members of the British Naturopathic and Osteopathic Association (MBNOA).

What to expect

Patients who go for treatment to a practitioner trained in one of these ways often expect that they will be subjected to some form of manipulation with the aim of 'putting a bone into place'. While this may well be the case, they are likely to find that manipulation is only part of the treatment, and possibly not even the main part. They may well find, for instance, that they are expected to participate actively themselves, by modifying their lifestyle and activities in various ways. The main aim of the treatment is to assess how well the patient's body is functioning in relation to the demands made on it by that person's environment, personality, and lifestyle. Having made this assessment, the practitioner can then offer advice about the best way for the patient to adapt and cope with the demands that are being made on him or her. Manipulation has a part to play in this, but real improvement depends on the patient's cooperation.

An important assumption underlying much of this approach is the idea that a great deal of suffering results from faulty use of the body – especially but not exclusively the back. Poor posture, especially in relation to driving, working, lifting, and sleeping can all cause strain on the joints and muscles, and it is believed by practitioners of manipulative medicine that this strain can lead to patterns of dysfunction that result in pain. Eventually this dysfunction can probably cause the kinds of damage that are detectable on x-ray, but well before this occurs there may be abnormalities in the muscles and other soft tissues that are not visible with present methods of investigation but are nevertheless perfectly real. Muscle trigger points (see pp. 23–4) would be one manifestation of this process.

Manipulation

Manipulation is used to help to break the cycle of misuse and dysfunction, although exactly how it works is not fully understood. The old idea that it somehow frees a 'stuck' joint is probably not correct; more likely it has an effect on muscle spasm that is limiting movement at the joint. There are considerable overlaps here with the way that acupuncture may work (see p. 72).

Contrary to popular ideas, manipulation need not be very painful or violent. Mostly it is gentle and pain-free, even in the case of the more vigorous manoeuvres. A wide range of techniques may be used: sometimes high-velocity thrusts, but often gentle massage-like movements to relax muscles, or repetitive joint movements to improve the range of movement of a joint.

The consultation

Practitioners begin by making a careful assessment of the way a patient stands and moves. Differences in the height of the hip bones and in the location of skin folds and other features can indicate abnormalities of various kinds, which may be due to recently acquired back problems or may themselves be the cause of those problems. Osteopaths frequently diagnose a short leg on one side or the other; the consequent tilt in the pelvis is thought to be a cause of strain on the spine. Sometimes the insertion of a simple lift in a shoe will give relief, although the explanation for this is not always obvious. Minor degrees of leg shortening are difficult to detect without the help of standing x-rays, which are not routinely taken, and even when leg shortening is present it need not give rise to any symptoms; the adaptability of the spine should not be under-estimated.

The way in which a consultation with an osteopath or chiropractor proceeds is quite variable. Some practitioners do not make the detailed assessment just described but restrict themselves to treating the main problem rapidly; in such cases a consultation may be over quite quickly. As a rule, however, there will be a preliminary discussion of your symptoms lasting five to ten minutes, a physical examination lasting about the same time, and then ten to fifteen minutes' treatment, followed by explanation and advice. Depending on your progress, further appointments might require repeated examinations on each occasion, or, if you were recovering well, there might be more time for discussion and advice about prevention.

Although it would be unrealistic to expect a dramatic and complete cure from just one treatment, there should normally be at least some improvement after two or three sessions. If no improvement at all has occurred by then there is probably no point in continuing with that practitioner's methods. Certainly, there is nothing to be said for continuing to have treatments weekly for months at a time, with little benefit.

Help for your problem

Practitioners differ among themselves as regards the kinds of problems they think they can help, but most would be prepared to tackle the majority of cases of acute and chronic back pain. There are some disorders in which manipulation could be actively harmful: for example, rheumatoid arthritis affecting the neck or a tumour of the spine. A properly trained osteopath or chiropractor would generally recognize such disorders and refer them for appropriate treatment elsewhere, but even the best trained person can make mistakes. This is one reason why it is generally advisable for patients to consult their family doctor in the first instance, because he or she will have all the relevant medical history and usually will be the person best situated to assess the appropriateness of physical treatment.

As a general rule, patients should receive somewhere between two and five treatments. After this most people are either cured or have reached a 'plateau' where further treatment produces no further improvement. At this point treatment should stop unless or until a relapse occurs.

Acupuncture

Acupuncture is a Western term meaning the treatment of disease by the insertion of needles. It originated in China and is probably very ancient, although the textbooks used by traditionalists today were composed in the Middle Ages or later. Traditional acupuncture has

68

a complicated theoretical basis. It forms part of traditional Chinese medicine, which is mainly concerned with the use of herbs; acupuncture is only part of it, and not even the largest part. Acupuncture has been known in the West since the end of the eighteenth century, and at times, especially in the late nineteenth century, it was quite widely used here; the modern revival began in 1972 with the visit of President Nixon to China.

Some Western enthusiasts have tried to adopt the whole of the traditional Chinese theory. This is a difficult thing to do, owing to the unfamiliarity of the ideas; indeed, the modern Chinese themselves are beginning to lose contact with these concepts, especially since the Cultural Revolution, and nowadays they are using acupuncture increasingly as a merely practical form of treatment without worrying too much about the ancient theories.

Western doctors who are interested in acupuncture, of whom there are increasing numbers, often practise it on the assumption that it works via the nervous and glandular systems, and can in principle be explained in scientific terms. There are some differences in practice between this modern approach to acupuncture and the traditional one, but mainly it is a question of theoretical assumptions.

Treatment according to the traditional system

Traditional acupuncture theory assumes that there is a subtle substance called *chi* that flows through the body in special channels, often called meridians. Numerous acupuncture points are thought to exist along the line of these channels, and the traditional acupuncturist tries to needle these points as accurately as possible. He or she also makes use of the traditional Chinese diagnostic system, in which changes in the quality of the pulse felt at the wrists is supposed to be very important. The underlying assumption is that disease is due to imbalances in the flow of *chi*, and the function of acupuncture is supposed to be to restore the flow to normal.

Ear acupuncture (auriculotherapy) is a variant of acupuncture which depends on the idea that there is a representation of the body in the outer ear (the auricle); the head is supposed to be at the bottom of the ear (the lobe), and the spine runs up the back of the ear with the feet at the top.

If you go to a practitioner of traditionalist acupuncture you are likely to be asked a lot of questions about your lifestyle, the aim being to see how far it is possible, in your case, to identify the causes of disease recognized by traditional Chinese medicine. The acupuncturist will then probably look at your tongue and feel your pulses. On the basis of this history-taking and examination he or she will decide which channels (meridians) need 'tonifying' or 'sedating'. Needles will then be inserted to achieve this effect. Usually quite a number of needles are inserted, perhaps as many as twenty or even more, and they are left in for about twenty minutes.

There are many possible variants on this outline. Some practitioners use electrical machines to stimulate the needles. This is obviously a departure from the ancient methods, although the use of electrical stimulation was in fact introduced by the Chinese themselves. In the case of ear acupuncture, needles may be inserted in the ear and taken out again, or in some cases they are left in for a week or so at a time.

As a rule the needling is not particularly painful, because the needles used are fine; however, some patients do experience pain.

Non-traditional acupuncture

Here the practitioner, who is usually a doctor, will take the history from a more conventional point of view. He or she will not use pulse diagnosis but, in the case of back pain, will search carefully for trigger points (see pp. 23–4) in the affected areas. This is an important part of the examination. Studies have shown that very many of the traditional acupuncture points described by the ancient Chinese correspond to trigger points recognized by Western medicine. Moreover, the Chinese have long known of the existence of 'occasional' acupuncture points that do not lie on any channel but which may become sensitive in disease, and these, too, are the same as trigger points.

If trigger points are found the doctor will probably insert a needle into some or all of them. This may be painful at the time, although not unbearably so; often the sensation is not exactly pain but something that Westerners find difficult to describe because Western languages do not have terms for these feelings. (Sensations of this kind are generally thought to be an important indication of successful acupuncture in both the traditional and non-traditional versions of acupuncture.) If no trigger points are found acupuncture can still be used successfully; the needles are inserted into those areas in which trigger points would be expected.

Many doctors practising non-traditional acupuncture make use of a technique called periosteal needling, in which an acupuncture needle is applied to the periosteum – the membrane that covers the bones – in the region of a painful joint. This is moderately painful at the time but it only takes a few seconds to carry out. Periosteal acupuncture gives particularly good results in many of the disorders associated with back pain. How it works is uncertain, but it may change the way in which the central nervous system processes and registers pain.

In many cases non-traditional acupuncture uses fewer needles than traditional acupuncture, perhaps only two or three, and usually they are left in for less time – perhaps only two or three minutes.

Which is better, traditional or non-traditional acupuncture?

It is impossible to give a conclusive answer to this question, because so far no comparative studies of the two approaches have been carried out. Another reason why comparisons are difficult is the perhaps rather surprising fact that, in some patients at least, it may not matter all that much exactly where the needles are inserted. The mere fact of having a needle put in, more or less anywhere in the body, will provide relief for a certain number of people.

Probably what matters most as a rule is not so much the theoretical assumptions that an acupuncturist uses as his or her own experience and skill. It is difficult for a patient to assess this in advance; all that one can do is to go on the recommendation of people whose opinion one trusts.

Is acupuncture safe?

Provided the practitioner is properly trained, acupuncture is a very safe form of treatment. However, since it consists in the insertion of needles into the body it can never be absolutely safe; dangers do exist, but they can be guarded against. To put the matter in perspective, the risk of a serious or fatal outcome from acupuncture is almost certainly smaller than the corresponding risk from taking a pain-relieving drug.

Many patients are understandably concerned about the possibility of acquiring serious infections such as hepatitis or AIDS from acupuncture needles. The great majority of practitioners today use disposable needles, which are thrown away after use; provided this is done there is no risk of transmision of infection.

Apart from infection the main risk of acupuncture is that a needle will penetrate an important organ, such as the lung or spinal cord. It

71

is essential that the practitioner should have a thorough knowledge of anatomy to prevent this.

How does acupuncture work?

In spite of a quite considerable amount of research in recent years, it is still not possible to give anything like a full answer to this question. There are, however, some pointers to possible explanations.

Clearly, it is unreasonable to suppose that acupuncture could remove disc material that had leaked out of a disc or reverse other abnormalities of that kind. Nevertheless, it can provide pain relief for patients who are thought to have suffered disc prolapse. Possibly this is because some of these patients have pain which is not in fact coming from nerve compression, even though investigations show the presence of disc prolapse – or perhaps they did have a disc prolapse to start with but now the pain is being perpetuated by other causes, such as muscle trigger points.

Inserting a needle into a muscle trigger point seems to inactivate it in some way. This may be a local effect on the trigger point itself, or it may be due to changes in the central nervous system (spinal cord) which 'turn off' the trigger point, so to speak.

Although acupuncture usually works best when there are definite trigger points it can also succeed when there are none. This may, again, be due to changes in the way in which the central nervous system works, or alternatively it may be due to the production of natural pain-relieving hormones called endorphins.

Perhaps rather surprisingly, suggestion seems to play rather a small part in the relief of pain by acupuncture. It does not seem to make much difference whether would-be patients believe in acupuncture or not – indeed, acupuncture works well in animals – but it is important that you should not be afraid of the treatment, because fear seems to turn off the response in some unknown way.

Training in acupuncture

In view of the possible dangers of the technique it is clearly quite essential that anyone practising acupuncture should be properly trained. At present there is no requirement of this kind in Britain; anyone at all may legally practise acupuncture.

There are several colleges of traditional acupuncture in this country. These award diplomas, which however have no statutory recognition. Some physiotherapists practise acupuncture, and there is an Acupuncture Association of Chartered Physiotherapists. An increasing number of doctors have learned acupuncture; numerous training courses in acupuncture are available for doctors, and there is a British Medical Acupuncture Society. There is no obligation for a doctor to be a member of the Society in order to practise acupuncture, and at present there is no acupuncture qualification for doctors, although some have attended traditional acupuncture courses either in this country or in China and may have obtained diplomas from those sources. Full members of the British Medical Acupuncture Society have attended courses in acupuncture and have built up a certain defined amount of experience with the technique; all are of course qualified in orthodox medicine as well.

Being treated with acupuncture for a back problem

It may be difficult to obtain acupuncture on the Health Service for back pain in some parts of the country, although many Health Service hospitals do now use it in pain clinics. It is available at The Royal London Homoeopathic Hospital, which accepts patients from all over the country and where there has been an acupuncture unit for fifteen years. An increasing number of general practitioners also use acupuncture and offer it to their patients.

As a rule, acupuncture for back pain would be given in an initial course of about three to six treatments; at first the interval between treatments might be one or two weeks, and this would gradually lengthen as improvement occurred. Eventually a point is reached at which further treatments make no more difference; at this stage treatment can be stopped for the time being, but further sessions can be given later if the symptoms come back – perhaps after two or three months or longer.

The success rate in back pain is quite high: about 70 per cent of patients can be helped to a worthwhile extent, although not all are completely cured. About a third of patients are unresponsive to this form of treatment. As a rule of thumb, if acupuncture is going to work there should be at least some improvement after the second or third session; if there has been no effect at all there is usually little point in persisting. Certainly, it is not justifiable to keep a patient coming for treatment for months on end with no discernible benefit, as unfortunately does happen sometimes.

All these remarks also apply to osteopathy and chiropractic, and this resemblance may not be accidental. It is possible that all these 'physical' methods of treatment work in much the same way.

'Acupressure' and other methods not using needles

Acupressure is a misleading term, it really means 'pressure with needles' and is often used to refer to the treatment of back pain by means of local pressure with the fingers. It is something that patients or their relatives can do to help themselves; it consists in firm pressure over the trigger points for one or two minutes, and it can be helpful; it is really a form of massage. But although it may give relief, this is usually rather brief, and it is seldom as effective as the insertion of a needle.

In recent years some practitioners have adopted the use of laser machines of various kinds to treat pain. This is supposed to be equivalent to acupuncture, with the added advantage that there is no pain and no risk of infection. Experience with lasers has been rather mixed; some practitioners have found them to be effective, especially in children, while others have not. If your therapist offers you this form of treatment there is nothing to be lost by trying it, but as with acupuncture you should not persist if there is no discernible improvement within a few sessions.

There are also various machines on the market which patients can buy to treat themselves without inserting needles. These consist of a battery-operated apparatus something like a torch, with a probe which the patient presses to a trigger point or acupuncture point for a few seconds. No proper trials of these machines have been reported, but most are unlikely to be harmful. Some patients seem to find them helpful, but because their effectiveness is uncertain it would be unwise to buy one without having had it on approval for several weeks first.

Non-physical alternative approaches to back pain

Although most patients will probably think first of some form of physical treatment (osteopathy, acupuncture) for back pain, it is also possible to look for a solution to the problem in a more 'medical' direction. The principal kinds of treatment here are herbalism and homoeopathy, which are not identical although some people are very unclear about where the differences lie.

Herbalism

The use of plants to treat illness is probably as old as humanity; indeed, it may be even older, for it seems that chimpanzees, our nearest living relatives, do something of the kind. Certainly herbal remedies have been used throughout history, and with good reason, for plants contain many substances that are extremely active when taken into the human body. Some of the most dangerous poisons known are found in plants, and so are some of our most effective drugs; penicillin, for instance, is produced by a common mould. Until the middle of this century almost all the medicines used by conventional doctors came from plants; examples include quinine, derived from the bark of a South American tree called cinchona, which the native Americans used to chew to ward off fever, and foxglove (digitalis), formerly used in country districts as a cure for dropsy (water retention caused by heart failure).

The main way in which modern medicine differs from the older practice is that it is based on sophisticated chemistry. From about the middle of the nineteenth century chemists began to develop methods of analysing naturally occurring substances, including herbal preparations, to find out what was in them and how they worked. This trend continued at an ever-increasing rate into our own time, and as a result there has grown up a huge pharmaceutical industry.

The general understanding today is that an effective plant medicine will have one or more 'active principles': chemical substances that are responsible for its effects. The pharmaceutical chemist tries first to identify these substances and then, very often, to change their structure so as to make them more effective or to reduce their tendency to cause unwanted effects. Sometimes existing plant substances are used as the starting point for synthesizing entirely new compounds, unlike any so far found in nature.

Herbal medicine, in contrast, makes use of the original plant without trying to modify it. Herbalism is a survival of the ancient way of using plant medicines. The whole plant may contain literally dozens of substances, not all of which have been analysed or tested by chemists; herbalists believe that using the naturally occurring mixture of these substances is safer and more effective than isolating just one of them and giving it in an 'unbalanced' way or modifying it 'unnaturally'.

Although herbalism is a conscious attempt to preserve the best of the ancient knowledge, some modern herbalists do recognize the need to assess their practice by twentieth-century standards, and to carry out scientific studies of what they do and how effective it is. New legislation about the quality and safety of medicines is also playing a part in this; in the past there was often little or no control over the way herbal medicines were prepared. And the question of safety is important, too, for contrary to what some patients believe, the mere fact that a substance is 'natural' does not guarantee its safety.

Very few herbalists have conventional medical training although some have undergone a lengthy period of training, but, as with other forms of alternative medicine, there is no statutory requirement for anyone practising herbalism to have had any kind of formal instruction. There is a National Institute of Medical Herbalists which maintains a register of approved practitioners.

A consultation with a herbalist is likely to include an extensive assessment of the patient's personality, lifestyle, and circumstances, because herbalists claim to tailor their treatment to the individual rather than to the medical diagnosis. In this respect, as in some others, herbalism has something in common with homoeopathy. The medicines may be given by mouth or they may be applied externally as ointments or poultices.

Homoeopathy

This form of treatment originated in the early nineteenth century thanks to one man, Samuel Christian Hahnemann (1755–1843). He was a conventional doctor who became (understandably) disillusioned with the medical practices of his time and cast about for something better. After many years of trial and error he arrived at the system which he later called homoeopathy, meaning 'treating like with like'. It has something in common with herbalism: most of the medicines in use in Hahnemann's time were herbal, but the principle of selection is different. The central idea of homoeopathy is to choose a medicine which, when given to a healthy person, produces symptoms as similar as possible to those of a given disease.

In the case of back pain, for example, a commonly used homoeopathic medicine is *Rhus toxicodendron*, or poison ivy. This is a plant that grows wild in the USA and causes severe itching and blistering of the skin in people who have become sensitive to it. When taken by mouth it also causes aching in the back and joints, so it is said to be 'homoeopathic' to both skin rashes and back and joint pain.

Another of Hahnemann's innovations was the use of very small doses of his medicines. At first he did this in order to avoid unwanted toxic effects, but later he came to believe that these small doses, when prepared in a special way involving repeated grinding

76

or hard shaking, actually made the medicines more active than they would otherwise have been. The great majority of homoeopathic medicines today are still given in a highly dilute form, and the dilutions are made in much the same way as that specified by Hahnemann. This process is called potentization or dynamization.

The consultation

As with herbalism, the aim of a homoeopathic consultation is to select the right medicine for the patient as an individual. A homoeopathic prescriber takes a detailed history, paying particular attention to the way the symptoms arose, how they progressed, what things make them better or worse, what time of the day they are best or worst, and so on. Importance is also attached to how the patient *feels* emotionally about his or her illness: depressed, weepy, angry, resentful or whatever. Many other things may be taken into account as well, although the details vary a good deal from patient to patient and also from prescriber to prescriber, for there are many different ways of selecting homoeopathic medicines.

In the case of *Rhus toxicodendron*, the features that might suggest its use would be an improvement in the patient's symptoms in response to warmth and initial stiffness and pain which wear off after a short period of activity. If there was an associated skin rash, for example in the kind of arthritis that can occur in psoriasis, this would be a further pointer to this particular medicine. On the other hand, flitting pains here and there, associated with a tendency to tearfulness, might suggest a different medicine called *Pulsatilla*, while a patient whose symptoms became noticeably worse in wet weather might be given *Rhodendron*.

Attention is directed, not only to the factors that affect the symptoms directly, but also the way in which the patient feels about them. The prescriber is likely to ask, for example, whether you feel anxious, or depressed, or irritable in connection with your pain. In some prescribing systems, although not in all, an attempt is made to find a so-called 'constitutional' picture for the patient, on the basis of his or her mental characteristics, reactions to weather, food likes and dislikes, and other things.

In mainstream homoeopathic practice the medicines are almost always given by mouth, usually as small sugar pills or powders. Sometimes one or just a few doses only are given and the patient is then watched for a time to see what effect follows, or else the medicine may be given two or three times a day for several weeks or longer. In mainstream homoeopathy medicines are given singly, but variants do exist; in Germany and elsewhere there is a tendency to give complex mixtures of homoeopathic medicines.

In mainland Europe there is a tradition of giving homoeopathic medicines by injection; this is also done in the case of a similar but not identical form of treatment called Anthroposophical medicine. A few practitioners in Britain also do this, particularly for back pain. The effect of giving medicines in this way can be difficult to distinguish from those of acupuncture.

As with most forms of alternative medicine, the majority of practitioners of homoeopathy do not possess orthodox medical qualifications. However, there is a long tradition of medical homoeopathy, going back to Hahnemann himself, and homoeopathic doctors having both conventional and homoeopathic qualifications are to be found in many countries. In Britain, the training of doctors is mostly carried out by the Faculty of Homoeopathy, a body incorporated by Act of Parliament. Doctors can attend courses run by the Faculty and may then sit for the examination to become Members of the Faculty (MF Hom.); some members go on to become Fellows (FF Hom.). There is, however, nothing to prevent any doctor (or anyone else) from prescribing homoeopathic medicines to patients, with or without having undergone any particular form of homoeopathic training.

Most patients requiring homoeopathic treatment seek it outside the Health Service. However, there are several hospitals in Britain offering homoeopathy within the Health Service; the largest is The Royal London Homoeopathic Hospital, but there is also a very active Glasgow Homoeopathic Hospital and smaller homoeopathic hospitals in Liverpool, Tunbridge Wells, and Bristol.

Diet

There are many popular books extolling the virtues of diet for arthritis, and back pain sufferers often ask whether they should avoid this or that kind of food, or alternatively should be taking more vitamins or other supplements.

In most cases the answer has to be that diet has no part to play in preventing or curing back pain. When the cause of the pain is a mechanical problem such as a prolapsed intervertebral disc it is clearly unreasonable to think that diet could make any difference. There is also no evidence that diet makes any difference to the rate at which the ageing changes in the spine progress. However, there are some exceptions to such generalizations.

Overweight

If you are seriously overweight (that is, more than 10 per cent above the maximum 'ideal' weight for your height), it is desirable for you to lose weight. The excess fat inevitably places more strain on your back, especially if the fat is concentrated in the abdomen or breasts, where it exerts greater leverage on the spine. On the other hand, there is no point in becoming obsessed by the question of overweight; middle-aged women, in particular, often find it very difficult to lose weight and keep it off once lost. Probably the best hope of doing so is to join one of the self-help groups that exist for the purpose; alternatively, the low-fat diet, in which not more than 25 per cent of the energy intake is fat (compared with 35 per cent or more in the average Western diet) seems to offer the best hope for weight control.

Arthritis

In the case of rheumatoid arthritis there is some scientific evidence that diet can influence the severity of the disease. About 5 per cent of patients with this disorder reliably report that certain foods make their arthritis worse; this group can reduce their pain by avoiding the foods in question. There may be more patients who could be helped by judicious avoidance of certain foods, but unfortunately it is very difficult to identify these foods; patients need to spend several months under professional supervision for this to be done. First, they are given an 'elemental' diet containing only the most essential nutrients, and then foods are introduced one at a time to see which make their symptoms worse.

This kind of dietary management is not suitable for patients to try unsupervised. However, a recent study from Scandinavia seems to show that patients with rheumatoid arthritis who follow a vegetarian diet, avoiding meat and fish but taking dairy products, generally experience a lessening in the severity of their arthritis. The effect is not striking enough for doctors to advise all their patients to become vegetarians, but any arthritis sufferer who is prepared to do so may find that it does provide a worthwhile measure of relief.

Medical or physical?

The physical treatments for back pain are in a sense more direct than others; they go to the seat of the pain. However, not everyone likes the idea of acupuncture or osteopathy, sometimes because they are afraid of possible complications. One advantage of the homoeopathic method is that it is almost free from unwanted effects; homoeopathic medicines are particularly safe. A disadvantage is that improvement, if it occurs, is likely to be slower with medical than with physical methods. In the case of acupuncture or manipulation one or two treatments are quite often enough to make a noticeable difference, but medical treatment often needs to continue for some weeks or even months before it becomes apparent whether it is helping.

As a general rule, unless you are strongly committed to a non-physical approach it is probably better to think of trying acupuncture or manipulation first. Of course, there is nothing to stop you having both kinds of treatment at once, and some practitioners may use the two methods concurrently; the disadvantage of this is that if you get better you don't know which has helped more.

Psychological and psychophysical approaches to back pain

This category includes a number of treatments that are difficult to classify because they are partly physical and partly mental. Some, such as meditation, concerned with reducing the physical effects of mental stress, while others, such as the Alexander technique, apply a psychological approach to correct patterns of faulty use of the body.

The Alexander technique

This is a system of postural re-education that lies somewhere between the physical and the mental. It is concerned more with prevention than with the treatment of acute pain. Its founder, F. Matthias Alexander, was an Australian actor who began to suffer from difficulties with his voice. He came to the conclusion that this was because he was inadvertently adopting an abnormal head posture during his performances, and this led him to study the way in which he used his spine. Eventually he formulated the system which bears his name.

Teachers of the Alexander method today tend to work in a variety of ways, but the general idea is that nearly all of us have unconsciously adopted inefficient or positively harmful ways of using our bodies, especially our spines; the Alexander teacher aims to restore what ought to be the natural way of sitting, standing, and moving. Initially this has to be done consciously, by continually giving oneself reminders of what one ought to be doing, but eventually the body adapts to the 'new' patterns of use and they become automatic.

Instruction in the Alexander technique tends to be fairly lengthy, and it has to be private because it is not available on the Health Service. If you opt to try this method, make sure that the teacher is a member of the Society of Teachers of the Alexander Technique (STAT) or the equivalent American or Australian Societies.

Relaxation and meditation

Psychological tension contributes to the pain of many back disorders, but especially so in cases of neck and shoulder pain. Many patients, particularly women, have noticeably hard shoulder muscles which are tender when pressed. This is often related to chronic anxiety, and in such cases patients may benefit from taking up one of the many forms of mental relaxation that are on offer today. It may be enough simply to buy a book on the subject or to listen to taped relaxation instructions, but some people prefer to attend relaxation classes, either privately or in Health Service hospitals, some of which offer this facility as part of the work of the Occupational Therapy department. Yet another approach is to take up some form of meditation; there are many varieties of this.

A simple meditation technique that anyone can try for themselves is just to set a few minutes aside each day to sit quietly, with closed eyes, and to allow the attention to rest on any feelings of strain or tension that there may be in the body. Five or ten minutes are enough at the beginning. The idea is not to get rid of the tension or to do anything particular with it, but simply to experience it and see what it feels like. One could think of the tension as a kind of message that the body is giving; a form of complaint, and the idea of the meditation is at first simply to become aware of this, without trying to push it aside.

If you do this, you will probably find that there is a great deal of tension in the muscles of your face, neck and shoulders particularly. As soon as this comes into your awareness you can 'let go' of it; your face relaxes, your shoulders drop a little. Before long your attention has wandered on to something else – perhaps some worry that you can't get out of your mind. Now check your muscles again: perhaps they have tensed up once more? If so, just let the tension go as you did before. Or perhaps you are now thinking of some quite neutral matter, and your muscles are still relaxed; in that case, you can stop meditating and carry on with your normal activities.

As you continue with this simple meditation on a daily basis you will probably find that you become aware of the tensing up of your muscles even outside the formal meditation periods; then you can let go of it immediately and so the cycle of tension and pain no longer builds up so intensely.

Exercise is another valuable way of reducing psychological tension (see p. 94).

Modifying attitudes: cognitive therapy

Although much can be done for many patients with back pain, there will always be some unfortunates who fail to respond to any kind of treatment, whether conventional or alternative. The temptation for such people is to embark on an endless quest for a cure; the next doctor, the next specialist, the next therapist, it is hoped, will have the longed-for answer. This attitude is usually a mistake. It is generally better to try to find ways of coming to terms with the situation as it is: not in the rather negative context of 'learning to live with the pain', but in learning to accommodate the pain without being completely dominated by it. This is the trend in some of the pain clinics run by anaesthetists in Health Service hospitals.

There are several reasons for this approach. One is that it may be possible to alter your perception of pain by changing your conscious attitude to the situation. (This is really connected with the new outlook on the way pain is perceived which was discussed earlier: see pp. 46–7.) Another reason is the idea that people who try to 'protect' their backs constantly by doing as little as possible may actually be making the situation worse. The muscles and joints deteriorate if they are not used, and if the muscles are weak the back is more prone to injury. Also, the absence of an adequate inflow of nerve impulses to the spinal cord from the structures in the back may increase the amount of pain that is felt.

At some pain clinics patients are taught specific mental techniques for coping with pain and for minimizing its effects. There is some evidence that these methods can set up a 'virtuous circle': the pain does not necessarily go away, but the patients are enabled to live fuller lives in spite of the pain. There are several ways in which this may be done, but the methods as a whole are given the label cognitive therapy. Although mainly used for the treatment of specifically psychological disorders such as claustrophobia, agoraphobia, depression and anxiety, cognitive therapy is also increasingly being applied to the problem of chronic pain.

Treatment may be carried out singly or in groups. The general idea is to get you to examine you automatic assumptions and beliefs about yourself and your pain and to change your behaviour so as to cope better with your situation. You are encouraged to undertake a programme of graded increases in activity. Psychological 'rewards' for pain, such as sympathy, are removed. Techniques for distracting attention from the pain are taught. There is evidence that this approach can be effective for many people.

Another helpful idea is for you to use a timer (a kind of stopwatch) to find out how long it is possible for you to maintain a particular position or activity without pain. Suppose, for example, that it turns out that sitting for more than twenty-five minutes brings on pain. You can then restrict the maximum time for which you sit to perhaps twenty minutes; the timer is set to this limit and will ring to remind you when it is time to move. In this way it is possible to anticipate the pain and prevent it from coming on.

Back treatment in pregnancy

As mentioned on p. 42 many women suffer from backache in pregnancy. Specific treatments for backache are rather limited at this time. Although some pain-relieving drugs are safe in pregnancy so far as we know, it is generally better to avoid all medication if possible. The same clearly applies to surgery, which would not normally be undertaken. Herbal medicines should likewise be avoided, since although they have been in use for many hundreds of years their safety in pregnancy has not been evaluated. Homoeopathy is safer, since the medicines it uses are generally so highly diluted, but even so their safety cannot be taken for granted, especially in the first three months of pregnancy (the most critical period). However, homoeopathy would almost certainly be safer than conventional medication.

Acupuncture is reputed to carry a risk of inducing miscarriage, and therefore should not be used, especially for back pain because needling the lower back is particularly risky in pregnancy.

Simple measures that can help back pain during pregnancy include getting enough rest and wearing an abdominal support. Exercises cannot be done in late pregnancy, but during the early months they can, and this will build a reserve of strength and tone in the abdominal and spinal muscles that will help to prevent backache in the later months.

6

Coping with Back Pain III:
Looking After Your Back

When you are young and healthy it is easy to forget about your back and to subject it to unnecessary strains that may be the seed of later trouble. Even when symptoms occur in a minor way, it is tempting just to ignore them in the hope that they will go away – as indeed they often do at first. And certainly it is important not to become a hypochondriac, constantly fearful that this or that incautious movement will bring on an attack of pain. The fact is that many episodes of back pain come on apparently 'out of the blue' or following a seemingly trivial event; in such cases the pain is probably the final stage in a process of degeneration that has been going on for years and about which little or nothing could have been done.

At the same time you should not be fatalistic about back pain; much can be done to prevent it. The possible ways of doing this fall into two main groups. First, there are precautions that you can take at home, at work, or during recreation, and second, there is exercise: both exercise in general, and specific exercises to prevent or alleviate back pain.

At home

Posture and furniture

It is well known that most accidents occur in the home, and probably many cases of back pain also originate in the home. But even before we consider specific precautions to take at home, it is sensible to check your own posture when standing and sitting.

Some people stand slouched, with their stomachs projecting forwards and an exaggerated 'hump' at the upper part of their back. This stance is more or less unavoidable in late pregnancy and for people who are seriously overweight, but even slim men sometimes adopt it. It results in undesirable strain in the lumbar and upper thoracic regions, and is an important cause of back pain – especially perhaps in younger patients; older patients have often adapted to their 'abnormal' posture and are unable to change it. If your posture is

85

defective in this way and you are under thirty, you should make a conscious effort to correct it, although it is important not to overdo things and go too far the other way. The military 'correct position of attention', with a super-erect spine, shoulders braced back and an exaggerated hollow in the lumbar region, is also undesirable, causing strain on the lumbar spine and aching in the neck and shoulders.

But the problem with attempting to correct these faults yourself is that your standing posture is so natural to you that any alteration of it, even to a posture that is anatomically 'better', is bound to seem strange at first. Indeed, you may well not be able to achieve this more desirable posture by your own unaided efforts. If this is the case you may benefit from advice from an osteopath or an Alexander teacher.

Sitting posture is also important. To a large extent difficulties with this are a reflection of unsatisfactory chair design. Most chairs, especially so-called 'easy chairs', appear to have been deliberately designed to encourage those who use them to adopt a poor posture. Sitting in them, we are more or less forced to slouch, with curved spine and head sticking forwards like a chicken pecking. To correct this as far as possible, place a cushion in the small of your neck and consciously bring your head back so that it is in line with your spine. In order to achieve this position you may need to place the television set at a higher level. For reading, your book should be propped up so that you do not have to look down at it.

When buying chairs, look at how far they permit the adoption of a functionally correct posture. Some back sufferers derive benefit from a radically different type of chair, in which they half-sit, half-kneel; the seat is angled slightly forwards and part of the body weight is taken by a second support below the knees. Those 'back chairs', as they are called, tend to be rather expensive, but they are worth looking into for anyone whose work or leisure involves them in a lot of sitting.

Your bed

The bed is another item of furniture that needs to be thought about carefully. It is sometimes said that back sufferers need as firm a bed as possible, and so-called 'orthopaedic' mattresses are marketed with this in mind. In fact, however, a firm bed is not necessarily the best for everyone, and some back sufferers find such beds uncomfortable. Certainly, it is not a good idea for the bed to sag, but a fairly soft mattress can be better for the back than a hard one. To quite a large extent, the choice of a suitable bed and mattress has to be a matter of trial and error, but the guideline to keep in mind is that the ideal is to keep your spine in as neutral a position as possible: that is, when lying on your side your spine should be more or less in a straight line. If your hips or shoulders are wide this posture may be better achieved on a fairly soft mattress than a harder one. However, the base of the bed, as opposed to the mattress, should not be sprung excessively.

Pillows

The number of pillow is, like the mattress, a matter of choice, with the guideline of keeping the spine more or less horizontal. For most people, two fairly soft pillows are probably best; they should be replaced when they have lost most of their bulk. Whether you use one or two pillows, it is important to make sure that you tuck it or them well under your neck, rather than placing the support just under your head and leaving a gap at your neck. Special horseshoe-shaped pillows are available to provide this kind of support, although you can achieve the same kind of effect with a rolled-up towel.

If you consistently wake in the morning with a stiff neck or a headache it is well worth thinking about whether your neck posture during the night is satisfactory.

Reading in bed

Reading in bed is rather difficult to carry out without straining the neck and back. If you lie on your back with your head propped on pillows you are liable to injure your neck, while if you sit upright with your legs in front of you there will probably be some strain on your lumbar spine. It may therefore be better to avoid reading in bed altogether, but if you find this irresistible you should at least change your position frequently, perhaps alternating between sitting with three pillows behind your back and lying on your side with a pillow under your lumbar spine to keep your back horizontal.

Sex

Sex can also cause back problems. Once again, the answer is to experiment with different positions to find those that are comfortable for you or your partner – perhaps with the help of a strategically placed pillow. A firm bed is best, perhaps with the mattress supported by a plywood board, and whoever is affected should take up an S-shaped posture, the other partner fitting into this as required. If any pain is experienced during intercourse this should be signalled at once. With a little experimentation it should be possible to find a position that is satisfactory to both.

Daily activities

Although back pain can sometimes come on after almost any kind of movement there are certain actions that are particularly likely to cause problems. The worst is probably bending forward and twisting the back at the same time, since this imposes a shearing stress on the discs at the moment when they are most vulnerable. Another dangerous activity is lifting a weight with arms outstretched, since there is then a strong leverage on the spine which has to be counteracted by strong contraction on the part of the spinal muscles. Avoiding these situations is largely a matter of taking thought and anticipating, but there are certain activities that should particularly be kept in mind. If you suffer from recurrent or chronic back pain, you need to think about all the things you do at home and at work, analyse them, and modify them as necessary.

Dressing

Putting on socks, tights and shoes can strain the back. Instead of bending down or standing on one leg it is better to sit down on a bed or chair. A long-handled shoe-horn will help with tight shoes, and shoelaces are easier to do up if you place your foot on a chair and lean forward against your knee. (Incidentally, this is also the posture described as an exercise for psoas stretching – see below.)

Hair washing, making up and shaving

Leaning forward across a basin to peer at yourself in a mirror places an undesirable strain on your lower back. Whenever possible sit down rather than stand, or arrange a mirror on an arm that will allow you to see yourself without leaning.

Housework

Dusting and polishing are generally light tasks, but try to avoid repetitive movements with one arm. Change hands frequently to even out the strain on your back.

The height of the kitchen sink is important. If it is too high you will have to lift things out of it at arms' length; try having something to stand on, but make sure that it is stable. If the sink is too low, on the other hand, you can reduce this problem by placing an inverted basin in the sink or by using a draining board across it.

When using a vacuum cleaner, especially a heavy one, change hands frequently and walk along with it instead of pushing it a long way away from your body.

Making beds can involve shaking heavy blankets or turning mattresses. Shaking blankets out of the window is a potentially hazardous task for the back. Get help with these things instead of trying to do them on your own.

Lifting

When lifting wet clothes out of a washing machine, avoid stooping; instead, train yourself to squat beside the machine. Ironing is best done sitting down.

Lifting small children is another potent source of trouble, especially at bath time. Squatting rather than stooping is again the rule, and avoid twisting the spine. While the children are still quite small it is better to bath them in a tub placed on a table than to lean into an adult-sized bath.

Lifting in general is hazardous. Always make sure that you have a secure foothold. Don't stoop, especially with straight or nearly straight knees. Get a good grip on what your are lifting. Always keep your hips lower than your head. Lift smoothly, without jerking, and turn with the weight by swivelling your feet instead of twisting your back. Finally, don't stoop to put the article down. Don't hold even light articles at arms' length in front of you; always bring them close to your body to minimize the load on your spine.

If you have to move furniture or other heavy objects, give some thought to the most sensible way of doing so first. Heavy articles should be manoeuvred onto low trolleys if possible before they are moved, but if this can't be done, at least avoid pushing them from their upper part. Usually it is better to sit on the floor and push them with your back or your feet.

Shopping

If you are walking back from the shops with a load, divide it into two and carry part in each hand rather than all in one hand; alternatively, use a shopping basket, although most of these are poorly designed and may themselves cause back strain. If you are shopping by car in a supermarket avoid over filling your bags; it is better to have many bags with fairly light loads than fewer heavier ones.

Gardening

This often causes problems, especially in spring when people resume work after the winter. Digging involves a lot of strain on the back, and so does mowing with a non-motorized mower. While doing these things, stop frequently for a rest and change of posture, and don't go on too long on any one occasion; stop *before* you feel tired. Weeding, although not heavy work, often causes people to stoop; instead, have a rubber mat to kneel on.

The standard design of wheelbarrow places a lot of strain on the lumbar spine. To avoid this, don't load the wheelbarrow too much; it is better to make a few extra trips.

In winter, be particularly careful when clearing snow, not only because of the lifting involved but because of the danger of a fall on a patch of ice. Clearing snow can be bad for the heart as well, because it entails isometric (see p. 99) lifting in cold air, which can alter blood flow in the heart muscle.

Home maintenance

The do-it-yourself enthusiast is always liable to find him- or herself undertaking tasks that may threaten the back. The main things to look out for are heavy loads, as usual, especially in relation to bending and twisting. Another kind of activity that often seems to cause difficulty, especially for older people, is any kind of work that involves looking upwards for long periods. Putting up curtains, fixing lights, and especially painting ceilings are especially hazardous; it is common for patients to say that after a few hours of this they have pain in their neck, shoulders or arms for several days or even longer. Moreover, if there is giddiness associated with neck disorders (see p. 34), standing on a ladder and looking upwards is potentially dangerous.

At work

In general terms the considerations that apply to back care at work are the same as those that apply at home. However, you may have less influence over the circumstances under which you work.

Naturally, the details of back care vary widely according to the nature of your work. The demands on an office worker are bound to be very different from those of someone employed in heavy engineering, and there will inevitably be some kinds of work that are simply unsuitable for anyone with a tendency to back disorders. But even work as seemingly innocuous as typing can involve a surprising amount of quite heavy lifting of papers and files, and of back strain.

If your work does involve lifting, remember the golden rule about not applying strain to a bent and especially a bent twisted back. If, on the other hand, you spend most of your time sitting at a desk, perhaps working at a keyboard, it is important to keep your posture in mind. The considerations here are the same as those discussed earlier in connection with sitting at home. Slouching is undesirable; you should aim for an upright but not super-erect posture.

To achieve this, the height of your desk in relation to your chair is critical. Much pain in the neck and shoulders arises because the desk is too high. It should be so positioned that your forearms are parallel to the floor. You should also ensure that you are sitting neither too near nor too far from your desk. If you have difficulty in achieving the right position you should ensure that you have a good chair that allows for adequate adjustment; some people find that the 'back chair' described above (see p. 86) increases their comfort considerably.

Even the best posture, however, is going to become uncomfortable if maintained too long. Every twenty to thirty minutes, therefore, you should move about, look away from your work, perhaps get up for a moment. Shrugging the shoulders often gives relief from neck and shoulder stiffness; also, stretch your fingers and perform the neck exercises to be described shortly (see p. 101).

If you have to do a lot of copying, don't lay the material you have to copy on the desk; instead, have it propped up in front of you so that you don't have to keep looking down.

Travel and recreation

Air travel

Travelling by air is liable to impose strains on your back. Even before you arrive on the aircraft you have to manoeuvre your luggage through to the check-in desk. It is best to have several smaller cases rather than one or two large ones, and to carry some of the load in each hand rather than all on one side. Once you have handed your luggage in at the check-in desk you should not be left with anything heavy to carry to the plane and you should avoid burdening yourself with heavy items, such as large bottles of duty-free drink. If you must carry heavy items as hand luggage, at least provide yourself with a portable wheeled luggage carrier.

If you suffer with severe pain or find walking difficult, it is sensible to notify the airline in advance and to ask for a wheelchair to be made available at both departure and destination. Airlines are generally helpful about this (and you may get through the formalities faster than your more mobile fellow passengers!).

Once on board the plane, you are likely to find limited room for your legs; accommodation is usually cramped, especially on charter flights. Again, if you notify the airline in advance they may be able to accommodate you in a seat that allows you to move more freely.

Especially on long flights, you should try to get out of your seat and move about from time to time – at least every hour. Remember to check your seat posture, and if necessary to ask the attendant for a cushion to place behind your back.

Driving

The vast majority of back sufferers – and, indeed, many people who do not normally have back trouble – report that driving a car causes them discomfort. There are several possibe causes for this.

The most obvious source of difficulty is the seat. Few cars seem to have seats that are designed to give the right support to the back – but even if they were, there are so many variations among people that it is impossible that everyone could find the same design of seat to be satisfactory. However, the commonest fault is lack of lumbar support, followed by too short a squab that gives inadequate support to the thighs. Unfortunately, a few minutes spent sitting in a car in a showroom, or even a test drive, are not usually enough to show you whether a given car will be comfortable for you in the long term. Ideally, you need to spend several hours in the car, but this is seldom possible unless you happen to have a friend who drives a car of the kind you are interested in. It is sometimes possible to improve a less than ideal seat by means of a cushion or a back support.

Your position in relation to the controls is also important. The height and angle of the steering wheel and its distance from your body can all affect you, and so can the height and position of the pedals. It may be possible to alter the angle of the steering wheel; the height of the seat can sometimes also be altered, or you may have to use a cushion if you are small.

A heavy clutch is a source of back pain for some people,

especially with town driving. In such cases it may well be beneficial to change to a car with automatic transmission.

A less obvious possible source of trouble is low-frequency vibration from the engine. This is a somewhat contentious subject, about which not a great deal is known; however, there have been some reports that noise of this kind can aggravate patients' symptoms. According to one source German cars are particularly troublesome in this respect.

Many patients experience pain and stiffness in the neck, shoulders and arms after driving for a time. This is hardly surprising, since driving, especially on motorways, requires that one sits in a more or less fixed position that may well not be the optimum one. Apart from making sure that your posture is as good as it can be made to be, you should also turn your head, relax your grip on the steering wheel, and shrug your shoulders whenever the traffic comes to a halt. On the motorway, stop frequently at service stations – at least every hour – and get out of the car to walk and stretch your muscles.

Not all the pain that drivers experience is necessarily due to faulty posture or badly designed seating. These factors interact with the psychological tension that so many of us suffer from when driving. This causes us to grip the steering wheel tightly and to tauten the muscles of our necks and shoulders; indeed, the tone of all the muscles in the back and in the body generally is probably increased. To a certain extent, no doubt, this is inevitable: driving in modern conditions is bound to be a stressful experience. However, it helps to counteract this if we make a conscious decision to improve our driving skills and to cultivate as detached an attitude as possible to the incidents that occur while we are at the wheel.

As with other load-carrying activities, it is important to take care when putting luggage into the boot or taking it out. Avoid using large heavy suitcases, and try to choose a car that does not have a high sill over which things have to be lifted. Remember the danger of twisting the spine when it is loaded, and avoid turning round to lift things out of the back seat. For the same reason, try to get out of the car without twisting your spine; train yourself to swivel your whole body round on your buttocks before standing up.

Changing a wheel is a potentially hazardous task for the back. The wheel nuts may be tightly done up; if so, don't pull up on the brace with bent back, but try to use your weight by stepping on the arm of the brace. (To avoid this situation, keep the wheel nuts greased and tell the garage not to do up the nuts excessively tightly.)

During the wheel change the spare has to be lifted out of the boot, where it probably sits in quite a deep well; get help with this if possible and avoid lifting with a bent back. Be careful, too, when removing the wheel that is on the car and when replacing it in the boot.

If you are a do-it-yourself enthusiast you may well find yourself peering into the depths of a car engine for long periods. This can place an undesirable strain on your lumbar spine; if you tend to suffer in this way it may be advisable to curtail your car maintenance or at least to divide the tasks into smaller sections so that you don't try to do too much in a day or a single weekend. Try to rest one foot on the bumper, or place a support for your foot on the ground near the car.

Exercise and exercises

Exercise is relevant to back care in two ways. First, there are the all-pervading benefits of exercise in general, and second, there is the use of specific exercises designed to improve the back. Although there is some common ground between these two ways of looking at the matter, it is best to consider them separately.

Exercise in general

There is an ever-increasing amount of evidence to show that regular exercise is important to maintain the health of the heart and blood vessels. It reduces the risk of heart attacks and it tends to lower blood pressure. In addition to this, exercise improves the strength of the bones and thus helps to prevent osteoporosis; it is therefore directly beneficial in the prevention of vertebral fractures. And exercise is one of the best ways of counteracting stress, tension, and mild depression; it is therefore useful for anyone whose neck and back pain is primarily due to muscle tension.

These benefits occur regardless of age. However, it is only sensible to take your age and general state of fitness, or unfitness, into account; it would be foolish to embark on vigorous exercise without preparation. If you are over 40, if you suffer from high blood pressure, diabetes, or any long-term disease of heart or lungs, or if you are seriously overweight, you should consult your family doctor before starting a programme of this kind. Walking, on the other hand, is suitable for almost everyone except those with very serious illnesses.

The choice of exercise is important. It should be something you enjoy, otherwise you are unlikely to keep it up, but some kinds are more beneficial than others. The best are those that involve large muscle groups: that is, the legs and back. These include walking, jogging and running, swimming, cycling, and dancing. Some games, such as tennis and golf, can also be beneficial, but both these may cause problems to back sufferers because they tend to involve twisting movements. Squash is potentially dangerous for the hearts of middle-aged people who are not very accustomed to it; it requires sudden explosive physical exertion and there is also a strong competitive element that makes for rises in blood pressure.

Whatever form of exercise you decide on, apart from walking, it is important to warm up gradually and also – equally important – to slow down gradually at the end of the exercise period. To change suddenly from rest to vigorous exertion is undesirable even for young fit people and can be fatal for the middle-aged or elderly; also, it can impose undesirable strains on muscles, ligaments and joints. You should perform stretching exercises before and after exercise to help prevent these problems.

In addition to these general precautions there are some specific things that back sufferers need to take into account.

Walking

This is usually the most trouble-free form of exercise; it requires no special clothing or equipment and can be combined with other activities. Even so, there are one or two things to look out for if you are a back sufferer. If you want to carry a load, even quite a light one such as a camera or field-glasses, avoid placing a strain on your shoulders or neck; if at all possible, use a belt so that the weight is carried by your pelvis, which is more rigid. Acquiring a dog may seem like a good idea to encourage you to go out, but the pull of a large dog on a lead can cause a surprising amount of back pain, so make sure that your dog is properly trained to walk on its lead. In much the same way, grandparents who take charge of a toddler for a week or two often find that this sets off an attack of back pain, from having their hand tugged about or from walking with a pushchair.

Jogging and running

Make sure that your footwear is suitable, especially if you exercise on pavements. It is worth investing in a good pair of running shoes that give adequate cushioning on hard surfaces; seek advice from one of the specialist shops that sell equipment for runners if in doubt. Also, pay attention to your posture while running; many people carry their arms too high, which imposes a strain on their upper back and neck. If you find that you suffer from neckache or backache after running, this is a sign that something is wrong with your technique.

Swimming

This is often recommended for back sufferers, with good reason. It involves movements of the arms and legs that are similar to those used for the treatment of back pain, and because the body and limbs are supported by the water there is much less strain on the joints and ligaments. (By the same token, however, swimming is less likely to prevent osteoporosis than, say, walking or jogging, because the effect of gravity is important for this benefit to occur. It also does little to control one's weight.)

The choice of stroke may be important for back sufferers. The crawl is good, especially if you can learn to breathe on both sides instead of only one, but not everyone is able to use this stroke effectively. The breast stroke is also good, provided you can learn to swim with your body in a more or less straight line, so that you exhale correctly *under* water, only raising your head to inhale as you bring your arms round. If you swim with your head out of the water all the time this may impose an undesirable strain on your neck muscles.

If you have difficulty in performing a good breast stroke you can swim on your back, which may indeed be the most beneficial position so far as your back is concerned. Finally, even if you can't swim at all, you can obtain a lot of benefit simply from moving about vigorously in the water in the shallow end of the pool.

Cycling

This can be a surprisingly good form of exercise for back sufferers. Some people find that they can use it even when walking is painful, and at least one study has shown that patients with chest disorders can get about better on a bicycle than on foot. Cycling has two main advantages over many other kinds of exercise: your weight is supported, and because you tend to lean forward the lines of stress in your spine may be different from what they are when you walk. Patients who suffer from narrowing of the spinal canal in the lumbar spine may find that they can cycle comfortably although walking is painful (see p. 41).

If you want to try cycling it is important to choose a suitable machine. Most people with back pain probably think that an upright posture will automatically be best for them, and therefore choose a 'sit up and beg' bicycle. However, this has the disadvantage that road shocks are transmitted up the nearly vertical spine, and although this can be counteracted to some extent by using a sprung saddle, such saddles reduce pedalling efficiency. A more sloping posture, of the kind provided by a 'sports' cycle, may therefore offer advantages. Dropped handlebars provide several different riding positions: your hands may be on top of the bars, on the brake levers, or on the drops themselves, although the problem then tends to be that you may have to keep your head in an uncomfortable position to look forwards. Fortunately, there are now various designs of cycle available that offer something of the benefits of both types: these are certain versions of the 'all-terrain' machines that have become so popular in recent years. Such bicycles usually usually have fatter tyres, which provide cushioning from road shocks (at some cost in terms of increased rolling resistance).

Whatever design of bicycle you decide to buy, it is essential to make sure that it is the correct size. If the frame is too small you will be hunched up, while if it is too large you will have to reach forward too far to grasp the handlebars. Both situations tend to cause backache and neckache.

Even if the bicycle is the right size you must make sure that it is correctly adjusted for you. Important points to check are the height of the handlebars and saddle. Handlebars set too low cause neck pain, especially with dropped handlebars; it is usually said that the handlebars should be level with the saddle or slightly lower, but if you have problems with your neck it may be better to raise the handlebars a little. If the saddle is too high you will rock your pelvis as you pedal, which can cause backache. The saddle itself should be horizontal, or possibly tilted very slightly nose-down; certainly it should not be tilted nose-up.

Dancing

Many people derive a lot of pleasure from dancing, and this can give good exercise. Some, however, do experience pain in the back as a result, and if that is the case you need to think about the kinds of movements involved. Young people who indulge in 'break dancing' – violent movements of the head – have on occasion suffered serious injuries to their necks, sometimes leading to paralysis.

Back exercises

Almost every popular book on back pain places a lot of emphasis on the value of specific back exercises both for cure and prevention, although the kinds of exercise advocated vary widely. Unfortunately, it has to be said that there is not a great deal of hard evidence that such exercises are truly beneficial, and still less about which kinds of exercise are best.

Indeed, there is no agreement about what exercises of this kind are supposed to achieve. The theories that have been advanced include relieving compression of nerves in the intervertebral foramina (see p. 20), shifting nuclear material away from a bulging annulus fibrosus (see p. 21), increasing the concentration of the natural pain-relieving substances known as endorphins, strengthening weak muscles, decreasing mechanical stress, stabilizing hypermobile spinal segments, improving posture and mobility, and increasing the input of pain-blocking impulses to the spinal cord (see pp. 45–6).

None of this means that back exercises are not beneficial, but only that there is at present no definite evidence one way or the other. So far as the individual back sufferer is concerned, the moral is that if you want to try an exercise programme you should certainly do so, but if you find the idea unattractive you should not feel that by neglecting to do such exercises you are necessarily imperilling or slowing down your recovery.

You should also keep in mind the fact that exercises can do harm as well as good. Those described here should be safe, but there are no absolutes in medicine and every individual is different. If you find that a particular exercise gives you more pain after you have done it, you should not persevere with it. A *moderate* amount of discomfort during the actual performance of the exercise is not necessarily a reason for desisting, but a masochistic 'going for the burn' (exercising to the point of severe pain) is certainly undesirable.

Types of exercise

Broadly, there are two kinds of exercise that can be used: isometric and isotonic. 'Isometric' means 'equal length', and refers to muscle contraction with little or no movement of the joints over which the muscle acts. 'Isotonic' means 'equal tension', and refers to movements of joints in which the tension in the muscles remains more or less constant throughout. If you pull as hard as you can against an immovable object you are carrying out isometric exercise, because the length of your muscles does not change although the force you are exerting increases progressively. On the other hand, if you hold a fairly light book in your hand and flex your elbow, you are performing isotonic exercise because the amount of effort you exert is much the same throughout the whole movement but your biceps muscle becomes progressively shorter as it contracts.

In everyday life most movements are partly isometric and partly isotonic, although one or other element usually predominates.

Many of the exercises advocated for the back are isometric, the idea being to use the muscles without damaging the already vulnerable joints by moving them excessively. This is probably a good idea in general, although one needs to remember that isometric efforts increase the blood pressure more than isotonic efforts, so that people suffering from heart trouble or high blood pressure should use isometric exercises cautiously and should consult their doctor if in doubt about the advisability of any particular exercise programme.

The general advice given to back sufferers is to embark on exercise gradually and gently, and this certainly seems the wisest course in most cases. However, there have recently been reports from Scandinavia of the successful use of vigorous back exercises to treat both acute and chronic back pain. In some of these programmes the patients perform, with assistance from one or two attendants, a series of increasingly energetic movements lasting for an hour or so, and involving perhaps eighty repetitions of particular movements with short rests at intervals. This method appears to have given very good results, but no studies comparing it with more conventional treatments have appeared so far. It is inadvisable for anyone with serious back pain to use this approach without proper supervision from a trained adviser.

Movements to avoid

Some exercises should be avoided by anyone with back pain and indeed by anyone potentially at risk of suffering from such pain, which includes pretty well everyone over the age of about 35 even if they have so far escaped problems. Toe touching with straight knees, and especially 'bouncing' in an attempt to reach the toes, place an unacceptable load on the lumbar spine. Sit-ups with straight legs and lifting the straight legs off the floor from the hips should likewise be avoided, since they hollow the lumbar spine undesirably. Neck mobility is certainly worth preserving (see below) but swinging the head round in circles is generally not a good idea.

Yoga

Yoga is an ancient Indian system for conditioning the body and mind. In its full form it consists of a variety of techniques for mental and spiritual as well as physical development, but most Westerners approach it mainly on the physical level.

The physical techniques of yoga are known as *asanas*, which means postures rather than exercises. Each posture is supposed to be held for a certain time. Some are very simple to achieve (one of them consists merely in lying flat on one's back!) but others, such as head stands, are extremely demanding and require years of practice to perform properly and safely. Most Indian yoga practitioners have done the *asanas* since childhood and are therefore very supple; it is quite a different thing when a middle-aged Westerner decides to take up yoga.

Provided the teacher is experienced and sensible, yoga should do no harm to back sufferers and some undoubtedly find it beneficial. But it is very important not to strain to achieve difficult positions, and some of the classic postures should not be attempted at all by the middle-aged or by anyone with a history of spinal trouble. This applies particularly to the 'shoulder stand', which forces the neck into a potentially dangerous position. Movements involving twisting of the spine should also be attempted cautiously or not at all.

Movements to do

The following exercises are safe if practised sensibly. They provide a mixture of movements to increase flexibility and to maintain and build up strength. Both are desirable, but in moderation.

There is no need to turn yourself into a Hercules of strength to prevent back pain. As regards flexibility, it is important to distinguish between limitation of movement imposed by muscles on the one hand and limitation imposed by ligaments and osteophytes on the other.

Adult ligaments have little or no elasticity and will not acquire any by being subjected to ill-advised attempts to stretch them in the hope of 'becoming more flexible'; this can only cause damage. Limitation of this kind is not necessarily a bad thing; indeed, people who are 'double jointed' – who have abnormally lax ligaments that allow their joints to move through an unusually large range – are particularly at risk of osteoarthritis later in life. Osteophytes, likewise, cannot be removed by forcing them, and they may even be protecting the joints by preventing them from moving excessively.

Muscular stiffness, on the other hand, can be relaxed with benefit. However, don't be tempted to stretch tight muscles by violent movements or by force; not only can this cause damage, but the attempt is counter-productive because stretching the muscle spindles and tendon organs suddenly causes messages to be sent to the spinal cord which increase the tone in the muscles and make them even more tense.

Neck movements

It is a good idea to take the neck through a full range of movements every day; twice a day is better still. Each movement should be taken to the point where it stops, either because a limit of the range has been reached or because of pain; no attempt should be made to force through the pain, but the movement can be held at the limit for a few seconds and then released.

1. Look up to the ceiling and down to the floor. (Repeat 4 or 5 times.)

2. With neck bent forwards, look to the left and right. (Repeat 4 or 5 times in each direction.)

3. Some patients with one-sided neck or shoulder pain experience

101

relief if the head is bent a few times towards the affected side. However, if doing this makes the pain worse, and especially if it begins to travel farther down the arm, don't persevere.

4. To strengthen the muscles in front of the neck: lie on your back on the floor with knees and hips bent and your head supported on two pillows. Then raise your head smoothly, bringing your chin down towards your chest as far as possible (this also stretches the neck). (Repeat 10–20 times.)

   Alternatively, sit in a chair and place your hands, with fingers interlocked, against your forehead. Without altering the position of your head, slowly increase the pressure against your hands and hold it for 2–3 minutes. (This is an isometric exercise.)

5. To exercise the upper joints of the neck, sit in a chair and, placing your hands lightly in your lap or on the sides of the chair, glide your head and neck from side to side four or five times like a Balinese dancer. (Not everyone finds this description easy to follow; try to get a physiotherapist to demonstrate it if in doubt.) This exercise should preferably be done first, before the nodding and turning exercises described above.

The thoracic spine

The main aim of exercises in this region is to try to maintain or improve mobility, especially in the upper part of the spine where many middle-aged and elderly people become stiff and immobile. An important way of doing this is to stretch the muscles on the *front* of the chest (pectoral muscles).

1. Stand in a doorway with the arms to each side and the palms against each side of the doorway, above the head like a Y. Keeping the elbows straight, press the chest (not the stomach region) through the doorway. This helps to relieve pain in the lower part of the neck at the back and in the top of the shoulders (yoke area).

2. For pain in the yoke area, try lying on the floor with a rolled-up towel under the upper third of the thoracic spine; the towel runs in the same direction as the spine. Allow the head and the base of the neck to fall towards the floor, and rest there for a few minutes. Also, and particularly while sitting, shrug your shoulders up towards your ears and hold them there for a few seconds.

3. To maintain movement in the thoracic spine and improve muscle strength, kneel on the floor with your buttocks on your heels; rest your forehead on the floor and place your hands, palm upwards, on the floor beside your feet. Starting from this position, raise your head and trunk from the floor to a horizontal position, bracing your shoulders back as you do so. Remember to breathe normally throughout, and don't try to hollow your lower back. Hold this position for a few seconds, and then relax. As the days go by you can increase the length of time you hold the posture; five to ten repetitions are enough.

This exercise can be made more vigorous if the hands are turned through 90 degrees so that the palms face downwards during the bracing back of the shoulders.

The lumbar spine

Throughout the day, whether sitting or standing, make a conscious effort to remember to check your posture. Try either increasing or decreasing the amount of lordosis; remember that there is no one 'right' posture, so experiment and see what is most comfortable for you.

1. While lying on your back with knees bent, simultaneously flatten your back so that your lumbar spine touches the floor and your pelvis comes forward; at the same time tighten your buttock muscles. This exercise can be done standing as well as lying, and should be performed at intervals throughout the day.

2. Lie on the floor and stretch downwards with your left leg as far as you can, tilting your pelvis at the same time. Hold for a few seconds and then relax. Repeat the same exercise with the right leg. (Repeat 5–10 times each side.)

3. Lie on the floor and bend your left knee and hip, and pull your knee towards your chest with your hands. Hold for a few seconds and relax. Repeat with the right leg. (This exercise stretches the psoas muscles; these are large muscles on the inner side of the spine that move the thigh.) (Repeat 5–10 times each side.)

4. Lie on your back with your hips and knees bent. Smoothly, and without holding your breath, raise your head and the upper part of your body off the floor and hold the posture for a few seconds; then lower them gently to the floor. (This exercise is to tone up your abdominal muscles. You can also practise turning your

trunk as you lift so as to bring each shoulder in turn towards your knees; this will exercise slightly different parts of the muscles.) (Repeat 5–10 times.)

5. Lie face downwards on a strong table; the edge of the table should be underneath your hips, and you should use a folded towel for padding. Grip the top or sides of the table with your hands, and then lift your legs and feet off the floor and raise them as high in the air as you can. Lower your feet smoothly to the ground. (This exercise strengthens the big muscles of the back.) (Repeat 5–10 times.)

6. Place your left heel on a chair or stool and, keeping your left leg straight, slide your hands down your leg as far as you can. Repeat with your right leg. (This exercise stretches the hamstring muscles – the big muscles at the back of the thigh.) (Repeat 5–10 times.)

7. Place your left foot on a chair, with knee bent, and your right foot as far behind you as you comfortably can. Keeping your right leg straight, lean forwards until your chest rests on your left thigh or comes as near to it as possible. Repeat with your right leg. (This is another exercise for the psoas muscles.)

Glossary

Ankylosing spondylitis An inflammatory disorder of the spine, characterized by pain and stiffness.

Annulus fibrosus The ring of fibrous tissue that surrounds and encloses the jelly-like nucleus pulposus.

Apophyseal joint see **Facet joint**.

Arachnoid mater (membrane) The middle of the three sheaths that enclose the brain and spinal cord.

Arthritis Inflammation of a joint or joints.

Articular Pertaining to joints

Autonomic nervous system The part of the nervous system which regulates the automatic functions of the body; it is divided into sympathetic and parasympathetic systems.

Cartilage A whitish smooth tissue that covers the bearing surfaces of synovial joints (qv); it is colloquially known as gristle.

Cauda equina (lit. horse's tail). The sheaf of nerve roots that runs down the spinal canal from the bottom of the spinal cord.

Central nervous system The brain and spinal cord, taken together.

Cervical To do with the neck.

Chronic Long-lasting.

Claudication Difficulty in walking (Latin: 'limping').

Clinical The features of disease that the doctor can detect with eyes and hands (clinical = bedside).

Coccyx The vestigial tail at the base of the spine, below the sacrum.

Connective tissue A network of fibres, made of a substance called collagen, and various types of cells. Connective tissue is found throughout the body; it acts as 'packing' and covers muscles, nerves, and other structures.

Dura mater The outermost sheath of the brain and spinal cord.

Epidural Outside the dura mater (Greek *epi*: on, outside).

Facet joint One of the small joints between the articular processes of the vertebrae. (Latin: facet = small face); also known as apophyseal joint.

Fascia A thin sheet of connective tissue (qv).

Femoral nerve A large nerve in the front of the thigh.

Fibrositis Strictly speaking, this implies inflammation of fibrous tissue – fascia. However, the disorder is not true inflammation (qv) but is characterized by localized areas of tenderness in muscles and other tissues; it is probably another name for active trigger points (qv).

Foramen (pl. foramina) (Lit. a hole). In the spine, the intervertebral foramina are the gaps between the vertebrae through which the nerve roots emerge as they arise from the spinal cord.

Idiopathic Of unknown cause (lit. self-caused).

Kyphosis Convex curvature of the spine; a degree of curvature is normal in the thoracic region but the term usually implies an excessive degree.

Inflammation A complicated group of changes that occur in response to infection and other insults. At the microscopic level there are changes in the kinds of cells found in the tissues and the release of various chemicals; clinically it is characterized by local heat, redness, swelling and pain.

Lamina (pl. laminae) A thin plate of bone (Latin: *lamina*, blade).

Ligament A cord or band of fibrous tissue (fascia, qv) that joins two or more bones together.

Lordosis A concavity of the spine; there is normally lordosis in the cervical and lumbar regions, but excessive lordosis represents a deformity.

Lumbago A popular term for backache affecting the lumbar region.

Lumbar Related to the lower back (Latin: *lumbum*, loin).

Motion segment A pair of vertebrae, with their associated disc and facet joints and also muscles and ligaments.

Motor (nerve) A nerve that supplies a muscle and causes it to contract.

Neural arch The ring of bone behind the body of a vertebra, composed of two pedicles, two laminae, the spinous process, two transverse processes, and four articular processes (two above, two below).

Neuralgia A vague term meaning simply 'pain in a nerve'; many kinds of back pain, especially those that are caused by pressure on nerve roots, give rise to symptoms that patients might call neuralgia.

Nucleus pulposus The jelly-like material at the centre of an intervertebral disc.

Osteoarthritis The same as osteoarthrosis; a misleading term, because the disorder is not really inflammatory.

106

Osteoarthrosis A wear-and-tear disorder of joints: it probably comprises more than one disease; sometimes only one or two large joints are affected, or the terminal joints of the fingers may all be involved, especially in women. (See also rheumatoid arthritis.)

Osteophyte An abnormal spur of bone that occurs in the spine as part of the wear-and-tear process.

Osteoporosis A disorder characterized by loss of calcium from the bones; it occurs particularly in women after the menopause.

Paget's disease of bone A disease, of unknown cause, in which the bones become thickened and distorted.

Parasympathetic nervous system One of the divisions of the autonomic nervous system, concerned mainly with the maintenance of the status quo.

Pedicle The portion of bone that joins the vertebral body to the articular processes on each side of the neural arch (Latin: *pedicle*, little foot).

Periosteum The membrane that covers the bones and helps to nourish them.

Pia mater The innermost layer of the sheaths around the brain and spinal cord.

Process A projecting piece of bone.

Prolapse The abnormal projection of some part of the body into an area where it should not be; in the case of the spine, it refers to the extrusion of disc material (nucleus pulposus, qv) through the annulus fibrosus.

Referred pain Pain that is felt at some distance from the place where the nerve is damaged.

Reflex An involuntary muscle twitch elicited by a stimulus of some kind, such as a tap on a tendon or touching a hot object; muscle reflexes may be lost if either the sensory or the motor nerve to the muscle is damaged.

Rheumatism A vague term; there is no such disease as 'rheumatism', but the term 'rheumatic disorders' applies loosely to rheumatoid arthritis, osteoarthritis, and other painful diseases of the joints.

Rheumatoid arthritis A disease characterized by inflammation (qv) of the joints but also changes in many other organs throughout the body.

Sacroiliac (joint) The joint between the sacrum (qv) and the ilium, one of the bones that make up the pelvis. There is normally very little movement at this joint.

Sacrum The triangular bone at the bottom of the spine, which forms the back of the pelvis.

Sciatic nerve The largest nerve in the body. It is formed by the union of several nerve roots in the lumbar and sacral regions.

Sciatica Pain in the buttock and leg in the region supplied by the sciatic nerve; also, by extension, in the region supplied by the femoral nerve (qv).

Scoliosis A deformity of the spine characterized by sideways bending; in practice, there is always a degree of spinal twisting (rotation) as well.

Sensory nerve A nerve that brings sensations of touch, temperature, pain and other sensations to the central nervous system.

Shingles Also called herpes zoster; a disease caused by the chickenpox virus, which is believed to have lodged for many years in the nerve roots in the spinal column and which causes pain and a rash in the distribution of the affected nerve or nerves.

Spasm Contraction of muscle that occurs involuntarily in order to protect the underlying parts from further injury.

Spinal canal The tube formed by the column of neural arches and vertebral bodies.

Spinal cord The projection of the brain that runs down the spinal canal as far as the lower border of the first lumbar vertebra; it contains both nerve fibres and nerve cells.

Spondylitis Inflammation of a vertebra.

Spondylosis The wear-and-tear changes that occur in almost everybody's spine with time.

Spondylolisthesis The slipping of one vertebra on another.

Spondylolysis Separation of a neural arch from the vertebral body.

Subluxation Partial dislocation of a joint.

Sympathetic nervous system One of the divisions of the autonomic nervous system (qv), concerned mainly with 'fight and flight' reactions.

Syndrome A group of symptoms that tend to occur together (Greek, running together).

Synovial joint The commonest kind of joint in the body, characterized by a capsule made up of fibrous tissue lined with synovial membrane.

Tendon A cord or sheet of fibrous tissue that attaches a muscle to bone.

TENS (Transcutaneous electrical nerve stimulation): a method of pain relief using electrical stimulation.

Thoracic Pertaining to the chest (Latin: *thorax*, chest).

Trigger point A point, or more often a zone, in muscle or other tissue which hurts when it is pressed and from which pain may be referred to other areas.

Vertebra (pl. vertebrae) One of the 24 bones that, with the sacrum and coccyx, make up the vertebral column.

Useful Addresses

The British Medical Acupuncture Society
Newton House
Newton Lane
Lower Whitley
Cheshire WA4 4JA
Tel: 0925–73727

The British School of Osteopathy
1–4 Suffolk Street
London SW1Y 4HG
Tel: 071–930 9254

The Faculty of Homoeopathy
The Royal London Homoeopathic Hospital
Great Ormond Street
London WC1N 3HR
Tel: 071–837 8833

National Institute of Medical Herbalists
9 Palace Gate
Exeter EX1 1JA
Tel: 0392–426022

British Chiropractic Association
Premier House
10 Greycoat Place
London SW1
Tel: 071–222 8866

Society of Teachers of the Alexander Technique (STAT)
10 London House
Fulham Road
London SW10 9EL
Tel: 071–351 0828

Index